AF808981

SOMATIC THERAPY
WORKBOOK
FOR MIND-BODY RESET

Books by Lulu Nicholson

Vagus Nerve Reset Workbook: Beginner's Guide to Polyvagal Theory and Simple Somatic Exercises to Calm Anxiety, Stress, Depression, and Trauma, and Improve Sleep, Digestion, and Nervous System Health

Anxious, Avoidant, and Disorganized Attachment Recovery Workbook: Apply Attachment Theory to Understand Your Behavior Patterns, Improve Emotional Regulation, and Build Secure and Healthy Relationships

Codependency Recovery Workbook: Step-by-Step Guide to Overcome Fear of Abandonment, Stop People Pleasing, Set Strong Boundaries, and Develop Healthy Relationships by Restoring Self-Worth and Self-Love

Transformative Shadow Work: Guide, Workbook & Journal—The 3-Step System to Embrace Your Hidden Self and Transcend Emotional Triggers & Past Traumas to Reduce Stress, Enhance Personal Growth, and Improve Relationships

28-Day Plan on How to Stop Being Toxic: Step-by-Step Guide to Boost Emotional Intelligence, Overcome Negativity, and Quit Destructive Behaviors to Achieve Inner Peace and Build Healthy Relationships

SOMATIC THERAPY

FOR MIND-BODY RESET

WORKBOOK

USE SIMPLE, SCIENCE-BACKED EXERCISES TO CALM ANXIETY, STRESS, DEPRESSION, AND TRAUMA, REGULATE YOUR NERVOUS SYSTEM, AND RESTORE LASTING EMOTIONAL WELLNESS

LULU NICHOLSON

Lulu Nicholson© Copyright 2025 - All rights reserved.

The content contained within this book may not be reproduced, duplicated or transmitted without direct written permission from the author or the publisher.

Under no circumstances will any blame or legal responsibility be held against the publisher, or author, for any damages, reparation, or monetary loss due to the information contained within this book, either directly or indirectly.

Legal Notice:

This book is copyright protected. It is only for personal use. You cannot amend, distribute, sell, use, quote or paraphrase any part, or the content within this book, without the consent of the author or publisher.

Disclaimer Notice:

Please note the information contained within this document is for educational and entertainment purposes only. All effort has been executed to present accurate, up to date, reliable, complete information. No warranties of any kind are declared or implied. Readers acknowledge that the author is not engaged in the rendering of legal, financial, medical or professional advice. The content within this book has been derived from various sources. Please consult a licensed professional before attempting any techniques outlined in this book.

By reading this document, the reader agrees that under no circumstances is the author responsible for any losses, direct or indirect, that are incurred as a result of the use of the information contained within this document, including, but not limited to, errors, omissions, or inaccuracies.

Contents

00.

Introduction

Healing takes courage, and we all have courage, even if we have to dig a little to find it.
–Tori Amos

“

When I was diagnosed with breast cancer, everything in my world changed overnight. Suddenly, my days were filled with doctors' appointments, test results, treatments, and an endless stream of uncertainty. My body became a battlefield, and my emotions moved through constant waves of fear, confusion, and fragile hope.

During treatment, I started seeing a therapist. Having someone to talk to made a difference; it gave me a place to cry, vent, and try to make sense of everything that was happening. But even after months of talking and eventually coming through it all cancer-free, I could feel that something inside me hadn't caught up.

My mind understood that the worst was over; the cancer was gone, and I was now a breast cancer survivor, but my body didn't seem to believe it. I was still tense, anxious, and on edge, as if I were waiting for bad news to come at any moment. I couldn't relax. I couldn't feel safe in my own skin. And no amount of insight or positive thinking seemed to change that.

That's what led me to explore *somatic therapy*, something I had only vaguely heard about before. I was curious about the idea that trauma and stress live in the body, not just in the mind. The first time I experienced somatic work, something finally clicked. I could feel what my body had been trying to say all along, and I knew I wasn't just talking about healing; I was feeling it.

Through gentle awareness, movement, and breath, I began to notice where my body was still holding on: the tightness in my chest, the knot in my stomach, the way I'd brace myself without realizing it. Slowly, those places began to soften, and I started to trust my body again.

Have you ever felt something similar, like your body was holding onto experiences you could no longer bear? Maybe you've tried to think your way out of anxiety or "stay positive" through pain, only to feel that no matter what you do, something deeper keeps pulling you back. That's because healing doesn't happen only in the mind. It happens through the body.

Somatic therapy teaches you how to listen to your body's signals: the tension, the fatigue, the racing heartbeat, and understand them as messages rather than problems to fix. It's all about restoring safety, presence, and connection within yourself.

Now it's your turn to explore this process for yourself. Whether you're recovering from illness, trauma, or the everyday stress of holding it all together, this work will help you understand and release what your body has been carrying. As you move through it, you'll begin to notice how healing deepens when your mind and body reconnect—when they start to communicate, restore balance, and guide you toward wholeness.

About the Workbook

This workbook was created to help you understand the connection between your body, mind, and emotions. Inside, you'll find simple, practical exercises that build emotional resilience and help you explore how your thoughts, feelings, and physical sensations are all linked.

To enhance your reading experience, I have included QR codes throughout the book to access guided audio versions of select exercises, offering you supportive voice-led instruction exactly when you need it most. Think of them as a calm voice walking you through each step, helping you stay grounded and present whenever you need a little extra guidance. This is your space to slow down, listen inward, and gently reconnect with the wisdom your body already holds.

Through real-life stories and relatable examples, you'll find tools you can start using right away to create meaningful change. The practices range from mindful breathing exercises to gentle movement techniques; simple approaches you can weave into everyday life. Each one is designed to help you reconnect with your body, calm your mind, and take charge of your healing in a way that feels natural and doable.

Together, these elements form a complete toolkit for healing. Each section is designed to guide you through your own process of transformation, using somatic experiences as a gateway to deeper awareness and growth. The goal is for you to finish these pages feeling more connected to yourself: grounded, centered, and confident in your ability to navigate whatever life brings. As you move through each chapter, you'll discover ways to create a sense of calm and build resilience, both within and around you, so you can better manage emotions like anxiety and fear that have held too much space for too long.

Preparing for the Journey Ahead

Before engaging with the content, I invite you to pause and check in with yourself. Notice where you are emotionally and where you find yourself in your healing journey. Take a few moments to reflect on the following questions:

What emotions might still be living in your body, waiting to be acknowledged?

Are there experiences you've pushed so far down that they now show up as tension, discomfort, or unease?

This reflection is important because it sets the stage for the work ahead. As you move through the material, you'll begin to map these feelings and transform them from sources of pain into pathways toward freedom.

As you continue forward, remember that healing rarely follows a straight line. Some days will feel light and full of progress, while others may stir old emotions or bring moments of uncertainty. That's all part of the process. Each step, no matter how small, brings you closer to feeling balanced, at ease, and more at home within yourself. Think of this workbook as both a guide and a companion, here to support you as you explore the deeper layers of somatic healing at your own pace.

Stay open-minded and patient with yourself as you move through the work. Give yourself permission to explore without judgment, trusting that each exercise and insight is a stepping stone toward greater emotional freedom. While some concepts may feel unfamiliar at first, with time and practice, they will become invaluable allies on your journey.

I wrote this workbook from my own healing journey, shaped by the lessons I learned through somatic work and personal transformation. My hope is that as you move through these pages, you'll reconnect with your body and mind in a new way, one that helps you release what's been heavy, build emotional resilience, and move forward with a deeper sense of ease within yourself.

So as we begin, take a deep breath and let yourself arrive fully in this moment. Think of this introduction as a gentle invitation to turn inward and recognize the remarkable capacity you already hold to heal, grow, and transform.

01.

Foundations of Somatic Therapy

Healing may not be so much about getting better, as about letting go of everything that isn't you— all of the expectations, all of the beliefs—and becoming who you are. –Rachel Naomi Remen

"

Healing begins with awareness, and one of the most powerful ways to begin that process is by learning to listen to your body. Your body is always communicating, even when you're not consciously paying attention. The racing heartbeat before a difficult conversation, the tightness in your chest when you're overwhelmed, the way your shoulders lift when you're bracing for impact; all of these are messages.

Somatic therapy teaches you how to recognize and work with these signals instead of ignoring or pushing through them. It helps you understand that emotional healing isn't just something that happens in your mind; it's something that unfolds through your entire being.

In this chapter, you'll learn the core ideas that make somatic therapy so transformative: how body awareness supports emotional regulation, how stored experiences shape your physical responses, and how reconnecting with your body opens the door to deeper healing and resilience.

Definition and Principles of Somatic Therapy

Somatic therapy is an approach that combines body awareness with emotional healing, based on the idea that your emotions are stored within your body. This type of therapy suggests that to heal emotionally, you must also address the physical manifestations of your distress. For this reason, body awareness becomes the cornerstone of effective trauma recovery.

Understanding somatic therapy begins with recognizing its emphasis on integration; your body and mind working together. Imagine your body as a library of experiences; each emotion has left its mark, whether through trauma, tension, posture, or movement patterns. By tuning into these physical and emotional cues, you can access deeper levels of self-awareness and begin your healing journey.

Core Principles of Somatic Therapy

A key principle in somatic therapy is developing *body awareness*; creating a conscious connection with your physical self and the sensations you experience. During therapy sessions, practitioners often guide you to notice your breath, areas of tightness, or subtle signals from your body. You might realize, for example, that anxiety shows up as a heavy feeling in your chest or tension in your shoulders. These sensations are your body's way of showing where emotional stress has been held.

Somatic therapy also emphasizes staying connected to your body in the *present moment*, a central part of emotional regulation and healing. This practice helps you notice how your emotions are influenced by your physical state and surroundings. When you begin paying attention in this way, small moments of awareness can create powerful shifts.

Consider a moment when you feel anxious and unconsciously clench your jaw. Noticing this pattern allows you to intervene on both levels; relaxing your muscles eases physical tension while also signaling calm and safety to your mind.

It's easy to get caught in thoughts about the past or worries about the future, which can pull you away from the present. Somatic therapy helps you gently bring your attention back to the present through simple practices like breathwork or mindful movement. You might take a few slow breaths and notice how your body feels in that exact moment. This awareness helps you respond to your body's needs with compassion.

Along with awareness and presence, somatic therapy also uses *sensory experiences* to support healing. Simple activities such as feeling different textures, listening to calming sounds, or visualizing soothing images can help shift how your brain and body respond to stress (Bishop, 2021).

For instance, running your fingers over a soft fabric can create feelings of comfort that ground you in the present moment. These gentle sensory experiences help your nervous system find balance and make it easier for your body to process and release stored tension and emotional energy.

In addition to sensory awareness, *emotional expression* plays an important role in somatic healing. Many people learn to suppress feelings connected to pain or trauma, which can create emotional buildup over time. Somatic therapy provides safe ways to express these emotions, whether through talking with a therapist, moving your body, creating art, or journaling. When emotions are acknowledged and released, you create space for deeper healing to occur.

The principles behind somatic therapy are meant to be experienced, not just understood. They guide you through the process of moving beyond trauma and into a greater sense of balance and strength. When you actively engage in somatic practices, you begin to change your relationship with the past. Instead of being defined by what happened, you start to recognize your resilience. This shift in perspective allows you to rewrite your story and reclaim a sense of choice and agency in your healing journey.

Somatic therapy is a gradual practice that deepens with time and attention. Some days the process may feel natural and easy, while other days it might feel uncomfortable or slow. What matters most is consistency, showing up with curiosity rather than expectation. Every time you bring awareness to your body, you strengthen your connection to yourself and expand your capacity to heal.

Scientific Research Supporting Somatic Therapy

In recent years, research has increasingly validated the effectiveness of somatic therapy, especially in trauma recovery. One landmark study involving individuals who were diagnosed with Post-Traumatic Stress Disorder (PTSD) showed that when participants engaged in somatic experiencing sessions over several months, they demonstrated notable reductions in depression symptoms (Brom et al., 2017).

Neuroscience is also shedding light on why this approach works so well. Studies now show that our physical sensations are deeply connected to how we process emotions (Giraud et al., 2024). When the body is given space to release stored tension, the mind often follows, allowing healing to unfold on multiple levels.

For example, when you're guided to tune into your body, you may notice subtle shifts in your emotional awareness or the way you express what you feel. This simple act of paying attention reveals something powerful: your body holds an untapped ability to influence your mental and emotional state. It's an area that traditional talk therapies don't always reach, yet it can be a key to deeper healing.

When we look a little deeper, somatic practices don't just affect how you feel; they also create real, physical changes in the body and brain. As your awareness of bodily sensations increases, your mind begins to shift as well. Research shows that people who regularly engage in somatic exercises often experience greater focus, clarity, and mental flexibility (Rapkoch, 2024).

Neuroscience explains this through the concept of neuroplasticity: the brain's natural ability to form new connections and reorganize itself. These changes highlight how somatic therapy supports not only emotional healing but also cognitive growth and adaptability.

Beyond easing the effects of trauma, somatic therapy also supports your overall well-being. By staying connected to your body over time, you can strengthen focus, clarity, and emotional balance in everyday life. This becomes especially valuable for people managing high-pressure work, big life changes, or ongoing stress, offering practical ways to stay centered and grounded through it all.

After my experience with breast cancer, I came to understand these principles on a much deeper level. The illness itself was traumatic; the diagnosis, the treatments, and the uncertainty that followed sent my body and mind into constant survival mode. Even after I recovered physically, I noticed my body was still tense, my breathing shallow, my nervous system on guard as if danger might return at any moment.

Discovering somatic therapy, and later learning about the research behind it, helped me understand why. My body wasn't betraying me; it was protecting me. Through somatic practices, I began to gently release the fear, calm my system, and rebuild a sense of safety from the inside out. Understanding the science gave me reassurance that this process wasn't abstract or imagined; it was my body's natural pathway to healing.

As more people and practitioners recognize how deeply stress and trauma live within the body, this approach is finding its place in modern therapy rooms.

Relevance to Modern Therapy

In today's world, more therapists are beginning to see the value of combining body-based approaches with traditional talk therapy. Many clients find that while cognitive methods like CBT, or cognitive behavioral therapy, help them understand their thoughts and patterns, something still feels unresolved on a deeper, physical level. Integrating somatic therapy bridges that gap. It gives people practical ways to calm the body, regulate emotions, and build a stronger sense of safety within themselves.

As our understanding of mental health expands, so does our recognition that healing is not one-dimensional. People are looking for approaches that consider the whole person: mind, body, and emotion, so the changes they make in therapy feel lasting and real. Somatic therapy brings this depth by helping individuals move beyond analyzing their pain to actually feeling and releasing it, creating space for genuine transformation.

This is where somatic therapy complements cognitive approaches like CBT. While CBT focuses on how thoughts influence emotions and behavior, somatic therapy draws attention to what the body is holding.

Our bodies often speak before our minds can make sense of what's happening, through tension, tightness, or discomfort. By tuning into these sensations with curiosity rather than judgment, clients discover another doorway to healing. Together, cognitive and somatic methods form a more complete map of recovery: understanding with the mind and releasing through the body.

Consider a situation where you are dealing with anxiety. Traditional therapy, like talking to a counselor, might guide you to challenge anxious thoughts. However, integrating somatic techniques, such as body awareness or grounding exercises, could help you identify and release the physical tension accompanying your anxiety. Through this blend, you benefit from a comprehensive approach that does not just treat symptoms but addresses underlying causes holistically.

The effectiveness of combining cognitive therapy with somatic approaches is becoming increasingly clear in modern therapeutic practice. Many therapists notice that when clients engage in body-focused techniques, they often reach emotional insight more quickly than through talk therapy alone (Orzechowska et al., 2021). Somatic methods act as a bridge between conscious awareness and the body's unconscious responses, allowing clients to access and process feelings that may have been stored beyond the reach of words.

Modern therapy benefits greatly from integrating somatic practices, as they open new pathways for deeper healing. If you've experienced trauma or PTSD, you may have noticed that traditional talk therapy can only reach so far. That's because some memories and emotions live in the body rather than in conscious thought.

Somatic therapy offers gentle, body-based tools to access and release these nonverbal memories within a safe, supportive environment, helping you reconnect with your body as an active partner in your healing journey.

The applications of somatic therapy extend well beyond the therapy room, offering tools you can use in everyday life. These practices can help you manage stress, tap into creativity, and build healthier relationships. The skills you develop through somatic awareness, such as grounding, breathing, and tuning into your body's signals, become practical resources you can draw on anytime. They support a greater sense of balance, presence, and emotional well-being in all areas of life.

By viewing somatic therapy as a complement to traditional approaches, we open the door to a more inclusive and dynamic model of mental health care, one that honors the whole person. This integrative framework respects your unique experiences and supports sustainable, long-term healing. Most importantly, it invites you to acknowledge your body's wisdom as integral to understanding and transforming emotional challenges

Key Takeaways

- Somatic therapy intertwines body awareness with emotional healing by recognizing that your emotions are deeply rooted in your physical self. The journey through these concepts highlights how tapping into the sensations and movements of your body can unlock a deep understanding of your emotional landscape.
- By building an awareness of how past traumas manifest physically and integrating practices aimed at being present and engaging the senses, somatic therapy becomes a powerful tool for reclaiming control and initiating healing.
- For you who are navigating trauma, anxiety, or personal growth journeys, the insights here offer practical ways to embrace the mind-body connection for deeper resilience and well-being. This approach empowers you to listen to your body's messages using simple yet effective everyday practices like mindful breathing and movement to nurture transformation.

Your path is unique, and by integrating somatic principles into your healing journey, you can create an approach that truly reflects your needs and experiences. Through this embodied work, you begin to cultivate genuine empowerment and lasting change.

In the next chapter, we'll take a closer look at how trauma shows up in both the mind and body and explore how somatic therapy helps you address these patterns with greater awareness and compassion.

02.

Understanding Trauma and Its Physical Manifestations

Our sorrows and wounds are healed only when we touch them with compassion. –Buddha

"

Understanding trauma involves exploring both its psychological impact and the physical manifestations that can persist long after an event. Trauma is a complex psychological experience where your mind and body respond to past experiences, often in ways you might not immediately understand or control. Your journey with trauma is unique, full of intricate connections between memories and physical sensations. Yet, you may not readily link this emotional turmoil to the aches and pains in your body.

This chapter invites you to explore these connections and consider how unprocessed trauma can manifest itself physically, urging you to listen closely to what your body is trying to tell you.

The Physiology of Trauma and the Brain-Body Connection

Trauma profoundly affects both the brain and body, often altering the way your nervous system processes and responds to the world. When you experience something overwhelming, your brain's neural pathways adapt in an effort to protect you. These changes can influence how you regulate emotions, respond to stress, and relate to others long after the event has passed. The imprint of trauma can shape your perceptions, reactions, and sense of safety in ways that may not always align with your present reality.

At the heart of these changes is the way trauma alters brain structure and chemistry. The regions of the brain responsible for memory, emotion regulation, and fear response, such as the amygdala, hippocampus, and prefrontal cortex, are notably affected.

The amygdala may become overactive, heightening anxiety and fearfulness; meanwhile, the hippocampus might shrink, affecting your ability to process memories accurately. This state creates a feedback loop where the more your brain is exposed to trauma, the more ingrained these responses become, making recovery challenging but not impossible (Rousseau, 2023).

The Role of the Autonomic Nervous System

Going deeper into this, trauma can dysregulate the autonomic nervous system (ANS), leading to an imbalance between its two branches: the sympathetic and parasympathetic nervous systems. Typically, the sympathetic nervous system prepares your body for 'fight or flight' responses, while the parasympathetic system aims to calm and restore.

However, trauma can keep the ANS in a state of chronic activation, causing ongoing stress-related physical symptoms such as increased heart rate, high blood pressure, and muscle tension (*How Does Trauma Affect the Parasympathetic Nervous System?* 2020). Over time, these symptoms contribute to a range of health issues, highlighting the necessity for approaches that soothe and balance your nervous system.

Stress Hormones and Physical Manifestations

Stress hormones are another piece of this puzzle. During a traumatic event, hormones like cortisol and adrenaline surge through your body, preparing it to deal with immediate threats. While this is necessary for survival, recurring or prolonged exposure keeps your body in a heightened state of alertness, potentially paving the way for chronic health problems. Conditions such as insomnia, cardiovascular diseases, and immune system suppression become more likely as your body struggles to return to a baseline state of relaxation (*How Does Trauma Affect the Parasympathetic Nervous System?* 2020).

Trauma doesn't just affect the mind; it can live within the body as what's often called somatic memory. This occurs when the body retains the imprint of past experiences, even when the conscious mind cannot recall them. You might notice unexplained aches, digestive issues, or subtle postural shifts that seem to appear without reason. These physical sensations are not random; they are the body's way of remembering. Somatic memories bridge past trauma with present experience, revealing how deeply the body participates in our emotional life.

Recognizing this connection between body and mind allows you to better understand and validate the physical and emotional symptoms that can arise from trauma. This awareness highlights why somatic approaches are so valuable; they help release stored tension, restore a sense of safety, and support healing that engages your whole being, not just your thoughts.

Instead of viewing trauma solely as a psychological issue, this perspective reveals it as a complex, multifaceted experience; one that calls for integrating both the mental and physical aspects of recovery.

Gaining an understanding of the neurobiological effects of trauma can help you make sense of your reactions and begin to normalize them. Many people feel confused or frustrated by the emotional and physical responses that follow trauma, without realizing these reactions are shaped by intricate biological processes beyond conscious control.

Viewing these patterns through a scientific lens helps demystify what's happening inside you and places your experiences within a broader human context. This awareness allows for greater self-compassion and supports the exploration of healing approaches that address both the mind and body.

Specific Areas in the Body Where Trauma Manifests and How It Feels

Trauma can impact specific areas of the body, creating distinct sensations and discomforts that reflect unresolved emotional experiences.

Understanding how trauma manifests in these regions is essential for recognizing its impact on your overall health and well-being. Let's take a look at some of the ways trauma can be felt in your body.

Chronic Pain

Chronic pain often emerges in particular areas, such as the back and neck, serving as a reminder of past traumas. This pain might manifest as persistent backaches that throb or burn, or tension headaches that feel like a vice gripping your skull. These physical sensations are not merely ailments; they carry the weight of emotional distress rooted in unresolved experiences, often resistant to conventional medical solutions.

Unexplained Fatigue

Fatigue can also manifest in the body, creating a heavy sensation that clings to limbs, particularly in the arms and legs. This profound exhaustion (which is often unexplainable) may feel as if every movement requires immense effort, transcending the ordinary tiredness that comes with daily life. This all-consuming fatigue is often attributed to the emotional burdens of unprocessed memories that drain your energy, leaving you feeling depleted even after rest.

Poor Gut Health

Digestive issues due to poor gut health frequently arise in the abdominal area, where trauma can disrupt normal functioning. You may experience recurrent stomach aches, bloating, or other gastrointestinal disturbances that feel unsettling. These sensations may be confused with dietary problems such as food intolerances, yet they signify the deeper emotional turmoil linked to past experiences. The gut, often referred to as the "second brain," reflects how psychological pain can emerge as physical discomfort in the abdominal region (Holzer, 2022).

Mobility Issues

Posture and movement are adversely affected by trauma, leading to a stiff or hunched demeanor that can be physically felt in the shoulders and spine. Muscles may become tense, creating a sensation of rigidity as the body adopts a protective stance against perceived threats. You might feel constricted, as if invisible chains are restricting your movements; a physical embodiment of fear and anxiety rooted in past trauma.

It is important to recognize that trauma symptoms can present differently in each person. While some may display clear physical signs like chronic pain or fatigue, others might not exhibit any visible symptoms, reflecting the unique ways in which trauma affects us. This variability emphasizes the need for personalized therapeutic approaches tailored to individual experiences and manifestations.

By recognizing the specific stress responses linked to your trauma, you begin to map your unique somatic landscape. Noticing where sensations arise and how they shift offers valuable insight into your personal mind–body connection. As you learn to attune to your body's signals, you develop greater awareness and control over your symptoms, along with a deeper understanding of how your trauma has shaped your physical and emotional patterns.

Case Study Examples of Somatic Symptoms

In exploring trauma and its physical expressions, it's important to recognize how past experiences can surface through somatic symptoms. These signs often appear subtly yet have a powerful impact, revealing just how closely the mind and body are intertwined. The following case studies illustrate this connection in action, offering real examples of how mind–body misalignment can manifest, and how somatic therapy helps restore balance and integration.

Sarah's Chronic Pain and Anxiety

Consider the case of Sarah, a 35-year-old professional who has been battling chronic pain for years. Despite numerous medical consultations, her pain persisted until she sought somatic therapy. Through this therapeutic approach, Sarah began to unravel the deep-seated trauma contributing to her anxiety and pain. As she looked into her past, she discovered unresolved childhood events that had trapped emotional distress within her body. The gentle process of somatic therapy allowed her to release these burdens, gradually alleviating both her anxiety and physical discomfort. This transformation sheds light on how resolving emotional and psychological trauma can directly impact physical well-being.

The Curious Case of Mark's Digestive Issues

Another illustrative example involves Mark, a successful entrepreneur who frequently suffered from digestive issues with no apparent physiological cause. His constant stomach upsets were debilitating, affecting his quality of life. Through introspective sessions with a therapist specializing in the mind-body connection, Mark came to understand that his digestive troubles were intertwined with emotional distress stemming from work-related stress and unresolved grief. By addressing these emotional triggers, he learned techniques like mindfulness and breathwork that facilitated his healing journey. This experience shows how deeply emotions affect bodily functions, suggesting that acknowledging and addressing these connections can build recovery.

Emily's Immobility: The Pathway to Emotional Freedom

Trauma's impact on movement is another area where physical symptoms manifest conspicuously. Consider Emily, who experienced significant restrictions in her physical movements following a traumatic accident. Her body was physically unharmed, yet she felt immobilized, burdened by an invisible weight. Somatic practices that combined gentle movement and emotional exploration helped her regain agility and a sense of emotional freedom. Through exercises focusing on body awareness and emotional release like yoga and emotional freedom techniques (EFT), Emily slowly discovered new pathways of mobility, both physically and emotionally. Her journey exemplifies how trauma can restrict movement and highlights the impactful changes that arise when these barriers are dismantled.

From Fatigue to Emotional Numbness

Fatigue is another common physical manifestation linked to unresolved trauma. John, a father of two, found himself constantly feeling drained despite adequate rest. Initially dismissing it as part of modern life's hustle, he later realized it was more serious. Engaging in somatic therapy, John uncovered layers of emotional numbness linked to past traumatic events. This numbness had been silently sapping his energy, leaving him perpetually exhausted. The therapeutic process involved tuning into his body's sensations, learning to reconnect with suppressed feelings, and releasing pent-up emotions. As he progressed, John's vitality gradually returned, a testament to somatic therapy's power to revitalize energy by addressing deep-rooted emotional scars.

My own experience mirrored many of these patterns in ways I didn't fully understand until I began studying the body's role in trauma. After my breast cancer diagnosis, I noticed how my body seemed to carry emotions long after treatments ended: the anxiety before each medical appointment, the tension that lingered in my chest, the exhaustion that felt deeper than sleep could reach. It wasn't just fear or stress; it was my body remembering.

Through somatic therapy, I learned to approach those sensations not as symptoms to suppress, but as messages to listen to. Gentle movement, breathwork, and mindfulness helped me uncover layers of unprocessed emotion connected to both the illness and the years of pushing myself beyond my limits. As I reconnected with my body's wisdom, I began to experience healing on a level that went beyond recovery; it became a reconciliation between my body, mind, and spirit.

These experiences, mine and those of Sarah, Mark, Emily, and John, reflect a universal truth: trauma speaks through the body until it is heard. When we learn to listen, we reclaim access to our own inner resources for safety, balance, and restoration. Somatic therapy offers a bridge back to that awareness, reminding us that healing is not something we think our way through; it's something we embody.

Key Takeaways

- Understanding the intricate effects of trauma on both your mind and body has been the central theme of our exploration. You've seen how trauma can disrupt brain function, leading to emotional and physical responses that become ingrained over time.
- The alterations in your brain's structure and chemistry highlight the interconnectedness of mental and physical experiences. Stress hormones like cortisol and adrenaline flood your body, creating a state of chronic alertness that can manifest in numerous health issues, such as insomnia and cardiovascular problems. This dynamic highlights the critical role of the autonomic nervous system and its imbalances, leading you to experience heightened anxiety, fear, and stress-related symptoms.
- The journey through this chapter also emphasizes the importance of addressing trauma holistically. Acknowledging and validating these physical symptoms as part of a broader human experience allows for acceptance and understanding. By demystifying your body's responses through scientific context, you can see your experiences as shared rather than isolated, encouraging you to seek out therapies that cater to the mind-body connection.

Believe it or not, your body is always communicating, sending subtle messages about your mental and emotional well-being. Somatic therapy helps you learn how to listen and translate these signals, guiding you toward the deeper roots of pain and imbalance. With awareness and compassionate self-exploration, healing becomes a full-body experience, bringing renewal and alignment from the inside out.

In the next chapter, we'll explore practical exercises to help you build and strengthen body awareness, one of the foundational skills in somatic therapy and a key step in creating lasting emotional balance.

03.

Building Body Awareness

Healing requires from us to stop struggling,
but to enjoy life more and endure it less.
–Darina Stoyanova

“

As you move through the demands of daily life, often focused on goals, responsibilities, and external achievements, it's easy to lose touch with the messages your body is sending. Turning your attention inward invites you to listen and respond to what you notice or feel beneath the surface.

At first, this inward focus can feel unfamiliar, especially if you're used to navigating the world through thought and action. Yet, the simple act of paying attention to your body can be deeply transformative, revealing both hidden tension and subtle sources of comfort that influence your emotional landscape.

In this chapter, you'll explore practical ways to develop body awareness and integrate these techniques into your daily routine. Through this practice, you can strengthen emotional resilience, enhance clarity, and cultivate a more grounded connection to yourself.

Introduction to Body Scanning Exercises

Building body awareness often begins with the practice of *body scanning*, a simple yet powerful tool in somatic therapy. This foundational exercise invites you to listen to your body's language, which often communicates through sensations of tension, ease, or neutrality. At its core, body scanning is a mindfulness practice; an invitation to be fully present and aware without judgment.

As you move through the exercises, you may notice areas of tightness, heaviness, or discomfort that you hadn't paid attention to before. These sensations are not only physical; they often reflect emotions and experiences held within the body. By observing what you feel, you create space for release and healing, while gaining insight into how stress, trauma, and daily habits influence your well-being.

To complete a body scan, it helps to follow a few simple steps. Below are five variations you can try at home or at work.

Mindful Breathing Body Scan

This method combines breathing with body awareness, making it an excellent technique for grounding yourself and enhancing your focus. By concentrating on your breath, you open up pathways to better understand your body.

Instructions

1. **Find your position.** Sit comfortably with your feet flat on the floor and your hands resting on your thighs. Let your spine be tall but relaxed, allowing your shoulders to drop naturally.
2. **Begin with the inhale.** Close your eyes softly and take a slow, deep breath in through your nose. Feel your abdomen expand as the air moves in.
3. **Exhale and release.** Exhale gently through your mouth, letting go of any tension you notice in your body. Take a few breaths like this, allowing yourself to settle into the moment.
4. **Bring attention to your feet.** Shift your focus to your toes and feet. Notice any sensations—warmth, coolness, pressure, or tingling. There's no need to change anything; simply observe what's there.
5. **Move upward gradually.** Guide your attention slowly up through your body—ankles, calves, knees, thighs, abdomen, chest, arms, shoulders, neck, and head. Pause at each area for a few breaths, noticing how it feels.

6. **Acknowledge and release.** As you encounter areas of tension or numbness, acknowledge them with gentle curiosity. Imagine your breath moving through those spaces, inviting softness and ease.
7. **Complete the scan.** When you reach the top of your head, take one final deep breath in and out. Before opening your eyes, notice any shifts in your body—perhaps a deeper sense of calm, warmth, or presence within you.

Progressive Muscle Relaxation Body Scan

This approach emphasizes the awareness of tension in muscle groups and the release of that tension. It's highly effective in making you more aware of where you hold stress.

Instructions

1. **Find your position.** Sit or lie down comfortably in a quiet space where you won't be disturbed. Allow your body to settle into the surface beneath you, feeling the support it offers. Rest your hands gently by your sides or on your abdomen.
2. **Begin with your breath.** Take a few slow, deep breaths in through your nose and out through your mouth. With each exhale, imagine your body softening a little more. Let go of any tension you notice in your shoulders, jaw, or belly.
3. **Start with your toes.** Bring your awareness to your toes. Curl them tightly and hold the tension for about five seconds. Notice the feeling of tightness, then slowly release, allowing the muscles to completely relax. Feel the difference between holding and letting go.
4. **Move through the body.** Gradually work your way up through each muscle group—feet, calves, thighs, hips, abdomen, chest, arms, shoulders, neck, and face. For each area, tense the muscles gently for a few seconds, then exhale and release. Imagine sending your breath into each area as it relaxes, helping it unwind further.

5. **Notice the sensations.** As you move through this process, pay attention to how each muscle feels when it's tense compared to when it's relaxed. You may notice warmth, tingling, or a sense of lightness spreading through your body. This mindful awareness helps you recognize where you tend to hold tension and how relaxation feels when it's truly embodied.

6. **Conclude the exercise.** Once you've scanned your entire body, take one final deep breath in, then exhale slowly. Rest for a moment in stillness, noticing the overall sense of ease or calm that's present. Allow yourself to simply be in this state before gently opening your eyes or returning to your day.

Guided Visualization Body Scan

Visualization engages your imagination, helping you connect with your body in a unique and immersive way. This method can significantly enhance relaxation and awareness.

Instructions

1. **Find your position.** Sit or lie comfortably in a quiet space where you won't be interrupted. Allow your body to settle into the surface beneath you. Feel the support of the floor, chair, or bed holding you. Adjust your position so your spine is aligned, and your shoulders can soften naturally. This is your time to be still, present, and connected with yourself.

2. **Begin with your breath.** Gently close your eyes and take several slow, deep breaths. Inhale through your nose, allowing your abdomen to expand, and exhale softly through your mouth. With each breath, imagine yourself releasing a little more tension. Picture yourself in a peaceful environment: a quiet forest, a warm beach, or any place where you feel completely at ease. Let this image fill your senses as you breathe.

3. **Invite the light.** Visualize a soft, warm light beginning at your toes. This light can be any color that feels soothing to you, gold, white, or a soft hue of your choice. As it begins to glow, feel its warmth spreading through your toes and feet, releasing any tightness or fatigue. Imagine this light as healing energy, illuminating your body from within.

4. **Let the light travel.** Slowly guide the light upward through your body, into your ankles, calves, knees, and thighs. Feel it melting away any tension, discomfort, or heaviness as it moves. Allow the light to rest for a moment in each area, soothing and relaxing the muscles, bones, and skin. As it travels higher, sense it moving through your hips, abdomen, and chest, filling you with warmth and calm.

5. **Soften and release.** As the light reaches each new area, imagine it dissolving any lingering stress or emotion that's been stored there. Let it wash through your arms, shoulders, neck, and finally your head. Notice how your breath becomes deeper and your body feels lighter. Take your time exploring this sensation of ease, allowing the warm light to reach the crown of your head and radiate outward, surrounding you in a soft glow of peace and safety.

6. **Rest in awareness.** Once the light has filled your entire body, rest in this stillness for a few moments. Feel the harmony between your breath, your body, and your mind. When you're ready, take one more slow, steady breath and gently open your eyes, carrying this sense of calm and connection with you into the rest of your day.

Sound-Based Body Scan

Utilizing sound can deepen your connection with your body, making it a fantastic method for increasing awareness and presence. This technique helps you tune into vibrations and sensations.

Instructions

1. **Find your space.** Choose a peaceful environment where you won't be interrupted; somewhere quiet, calm, and comfortable. Sit or lie down in a relaxed position, letting your body settle into the surface beneath you. Take a few deep breaths to signal to your body that it's time to slow down and listen.

2. **Begin with listening.** Close your eyes and bring your attention to the sounds around you. Notice the layers of sound, the distant hum of traffic, the rustle of leaves, the rhythm of your own breath, or perhaps gentle music or a singing bowl if you're using one. Try not to label or judge what you hear; simply let the sounds exist, flowing naturally in and out of your awareness.

3. **Connect sound with sensation.** Gradually begin to shift your focus from external hearing to internal feeling. Notice how the sounds interact with your body. Can you sense a vibration, a pulse, or a subtle shift in energy? Observe how sound moves through you, perhaps your chest rises and falls with your breath, or you feel a quiet hum in your fingertips or spine.

4. **Move through the body.** Bring your attention to your toes and slowly move upward: feet, calves, thighs, abdomen, chest, arms, shoulders, neck, and head. As you move through each area, notice whether the sounds evoke any sensations there. Some areas may feel more alive, others quieter or heavier. Allow yourself to simply notice without trying to change anything.

5. **Let the sound wash through you.** Imagine each sound gently flowing over and through you like waves of vibration. Let this experience heighten your awareness of your body's rhythms and presence. Feel how sound connects you to the moment, anchoring you in your senses, calming your mind, and deepening your connection to the space within and around you.

6. **Rest in stillness.** When you feel ready, take a few slow breaths and sit quietly for a moment. Notice any changes in your body, perhaps a sense of openness, ease, or calm. When you open your eyes, carry that sense of grounded awareness with you as you move back into your day.

Movement-Based Body Scan

Engaging in gentle movements while practicing body awareness can enhance the experience. This method helps you recognize sensations and embrace them through action.

Instructions

1. **Prepare your space.** Choose a quiet, open area where you can move freely without distractions. Make sure the lighting feels comfortable and the temperature suits you. Stand barefoot if possible, allowing your feet to make full contact with the ground. Take a few moments to simply arrive, letting go of external thoughts or expectations as you center yourself in the present moment.

2. **Find your grounding.** Stand tall with your feet hip-width apart, knees slightly soft, and shoulders relaxed. Feel the weight of your body evenly distributed between both feet. Take a slow, deep breath in through your nose, sensing your connection with the floor beneath you. As you exhale, imagine any tension draining downward through your feet into the earth, leaving you steady and grounded.

3. **Begin with breath and movement.** Slowly raise your arms above your head as you inhale deeply, stretching gently toward the sky. Notice the expansion in your ribs and the lengthening through your spine. As you exhale, lower your arms slowly to your sides, feeling your body release into the rhythm of your breath. Continue this movement a few times, allowing the flow of breath and motion to become one seamless rhythm.

4. **Bring awareness to each part of your body.** As you continue moving, direct your attention to specific parts of your body, starting with your feet. Notice how they anchor you and support your weight. Gradually shift your focus upward, through your legs, hips, abdomen, chest, shoulders, arms, neck, and head, observing how each part feels as it moves. Pay attention to sensations of warmth, tightness, ease, or energy flow without trying to change them.

5. **Introduce gentle variations.** Incorporate slow stretches, twists, or side bends as they feel natural. You might rotate your shoulders, circle your wrists, or sway gently from side to side. Let your body guide the movement, keeping it fluid and intuitive rather than structured. Imagine each motion creating space inside you, releasing stored tension and awakening vitality throughout your system.

6. **Pause and integrate.** When you're ready, bring your movements to a gradual stop. Stand still with your arms at your sides and your eyes closed or softly focused. Take a few deep breaths and notice the sensations pulsing through your body, the heartbeat, warmth, and subtle energy this movement has awakened. Feel yourself grounded, open, and fully present in your body before returning to your day.

Tuning In:
Strengthening Your Inner Awareness

At any moment, your body is sending messages: your heartbeat quickening, your breath deepening, your stomach tightening, or your muscles softening. This inner communication is part of what's known as *interoception*, the sense that helps you perceive what's happening inside your body (Schmitt & Schoen, 2022). It acts as an internal compass, guiding you toward balance and helping you understand your emotional landscape amid life's many demands.

Developing this inner awareness is important in managing anxiety and supporting trauma recovery. When you learn to tune in to your body's signals, your pulse, breathing rhythm, or hunger cues, you begin to recognize how your system responds to stress, fear, or calm. This awareness helps you regulate emotions more effectively and respond to challenges from a grounded, centered place. It becomes a bridge between body and mind, offering stability even when external circumstances feel uncertain.

You can strengthen this connection through simple, daily practices that increase your sensitivity to internal cues and help you feel more at home in your body. The following exercises are designed to guide you in building this awareness gently and consistently.

Feelings and Flavors

This exercise blends mindfulness with the simple act of eating, helping you tune in to your body's sensations and responses to taste, texture, and satisfaction. It encourages you to slow down, savor each bite, and notice how food affects your physical and emotional state. The following steps will guide you through this mindful eating practice.

Steps

1. Next time you prepare to have a meal, choose something new or complex in flavor (like dark chocolate or a fresh fruit).
2. Before eating, take a moment to observe the food: its colors, texture, and smell.
3. Take a small bite and allow the food to rest on your tongue. Notice the initial sensations.
4. As you chew, pay attention to the different flavors that emerge. Note how they change with each bite.
5. Reflect on how your body feels as you eat. Are you hungry, satisfied, or full?
6. After finishing, reflect on your experience, focusing on the sensations and emotions that arose during the exercise.

____

____

____

____

____

____

Emotion Mapping

This activity helps you explore the connection between your emotions and the physical sensations that accompany them, deepening your interoceptive awareness. By noticing where and how emotions show up in your body, you begin to understand your inner experience on a more intuitive level. The following guidelines will help you get started with this reflective practice.

Steps

1. Find a quiet space and sit in a comfortable position.
2. Take a few deep breaths to relax your body and mind.
3. Recall a recent experience that triggered a strong emotion (e.g., joy, anger, or sadness).
4. Close your eyes and visualize that moment, allowing the feelings to resurface.
5. While experiencing the emotion, note the physical sensations that arise: do you feel tightness in your chest, butterflies in your stomach, or warmth in your cheeks?
6. Visualizing your emotions on a body map, marking where certain feelings arise and using colors or symbols to represent them, can bring deeper awareness to your inner experience.
7. Afterward, reflect on the connections between your physical sensations and emotional responses.

Breath Awareness Walk

This exercise combines gentle movement with mindful breathing, helping you connect more deeply with your body as you walk. It encourages you to notice the rhythm of your breath, the sensations in your muscles, and the way your body moves through space, allowing a sense of calm and presence to naturally emerge with each step.

Steps

1. Choose a place to walk, preferably in nature or a quiet area where you can focus.
2. Begin walking at a natural pace, and take a moment to notice your surroundings—the colors, sounds, and smells.
3. As you walk, shift your focus to your breath. Notice how it changes with each step.
4. Count your steps for every inhale and exhale (e.g., inhale for four steps, exhale for four steps).
5. If your mind wanders, gently bring your attention back to your breath and the sensations in your body as you walk.
6. After 10–15 minutes, find a spot to sit quietly and reflect on how the walk affected your awareness of your body and your surroundings.
7. Journal about this experience, detailing any changes in your bodily sensations during the walk.

The Sensory Journal

Keeping a sensory journal helps you notice and reflect on your bodily sensations over time, deepening your connection to interoceptive awareness. This practice invites you to slow down, tune in to your body's subtle cues, and observe how your physical sensations shift in response to emotions, environments, and daily experiences. Try the following steps next time you tune in to your body's sensations and want to explore them more deeply.

Steps

1. At the end of each day, set aside 10–15 minutes to reflect on your bodily sensations throughout the day.
2. Notice specific moments when you felt a strong sensation (e.g., hunger, fatigue, stress, excitement).
3. For each moment, describe how the sensation felt physically. Use descriptive language—was it sharp, dull, prickly, or warm?
4. Note any thoughts or emotions that arose with these sensations.
5. Every week, review your observations to identify patterns and triggers related to your bodily sensations.
6. Consider setting intentions for the following week based on your reflections, such as practicing more mindfulness or taking breaks when necessary.

Techniques for Grounding

Grounding techniques help you create a sense of safety and presence, especially when recovering from trauma or managing anxiety. During moments of emotional intensity, these practices provide stability and remind your body that it is safe in the here and now.

By anchoring yourself in the present moment, you can interrupt spiraling thoughts or distressing memories and return to a calmer, more centered state (Caporuscio, 2024). This state of presence becomes the foundation for healing, offering a mental and emotional space where your system can begin to rest and recover.

Grounding became one of the most meaningful tools in my own healing. When everything in my life felt uncertain, I often turned to simple practices that reconnected me with the present moment, especially nature, touch, and breath. These moments reminded me that safety could be rebuilt from the inside out.

The following are a few grounding practices you can explore to help you reconnect with your body and cultivate a greater sense of calm.

Nature's Touch

This grounding exercise invites you to immerse yourself in the healing presence of nature and connect with the world through your senses. By tuning into the textures, temperatures, and sounds around you, you begin to feel supported by the natural environment. Engaging with these physical sensations, whether it's the earth beneath your feet, the wind on your skin, or sunlight on your face, helps calm the mind and restore a sense of balance within.

Instructions

1. Find a quiet outdoor space, such as a park or garden, where you can sit comfortably.
2. Close your eyes and take a few deep breaths, allowing yourself to fully relax.
3. Reach out and touch the grass, soil, or the bark of a tree. As you are doing so, pay attention to the texture and temperature.

4. Focus on the feelings of the ground beneath you and the natural elements around you. If possible, take off your shoes and feel the earth with your feet.
5. Stay in this moment for at least 5 minutes and allow nature to ground you.

Sensory Scavenger Hunt

This interactive grounding activity helps you engage your senses and shift your focus away from intrusive thoughts. A sensory scavenger hunt invites you to explore your surroundings with curiosity and presence, using sight, sound, touch, smell, and even taste to reconnect with the here and now. By intentionally noticing the details of your environment, you anchor yourself in the present moment and give your nervous system a chance to settle and reset.

Instructions

1. Challenge yourself to find three items for each sense in your environment: sight, sound, touch, taste, and smell.
2. For sight, look for colors, shapes, or patterns. For sound, listen for natural or mechanical noises. For touch, find items with different textures.
3. For taste, if applicable, focus on any food or drinks you have nearby. For smell, identify scents in the air or those around you.
4. Reflect on the experience by noting what you found and how it made you feel.

Breath of Colors

Channel the calming properties of colors through mindful breathing. This technique allows you to visualize and breathe in colors that evoke comfort and peace, helping you to reconnect with yourself.

Instructions

1. **Settle into stillness.** Find a quiet, comfortable space where you won't be disturbed. Sit or lie down in a position that allows your body to relax fully. Feel the surface beneath you supporting your weight and take a moment to let your body arrive in the present.
2. **Begin with the breath.** Gently close your eyes and take a few deep, slow breaths. Inhale through your nose and exhale through your mouth. With each exhale, imagine tension leaving your body, your shoulders dropping, your jaw softening, and your chest loosening.
3. **Select your color.** Bring to mind a color that feels soothing or uplifting to you. It could be blue for tranquility, green for renewal, pink for compassion, or any shade that feels comforting. Trust your instinct; your body often knows what color it needs.

4. **Visualize the color surrounding you.** Picture this color forming a soft, radiant light around your body. With each inhale, imagine the light growing stronger and brighter, filling you with warmth, ease, and a deep sense of safety. Let it move gently through you, from your toes to the crown of your head, illuminating every cell with calm.
5. **Release with the exhale.** As you exhale through your mouth, visualize any distressing thoughts, emotions, or memories leaving your body as a different color, perhaps gray, black, or a muted tone. Watch this color fade and dissolve into the air, taking the heaviness with it.
6. **Continue the cycle.** Repeat this process for several minutes, inhaling your healing color and exhaling the color of release. Focus on the rhythm of your breath and the gentle movement of color flowing in and out. Allow yourself to rest in this experience of lightness and peace.
7. **Return with gratitude.** When you feel complete, take one last deep breath and imagine both colors blending into a soft glow of balance. Slowly open your eyes and notice how your body feels, perhaps a little lighter, calmer, or more grounded. Take a moment to thank yourself for showing up to this practice.

The Emotion Ocean

Ride the waves of your emotions with this metaphorical grounding technique. By picturing your feelings as ocean waves, you can learn to observe and manage them rather than be overwhelmed by them.

Instructions

1. **Find your position.** Sit or lie down in a comfortable place where you can relax without distractions. Allow your body to settle into the surface beneath you. Let your shoulders drop and your hands rest gently by your sides or on your abdomen. When you're ready, softly close your eyes and take a few slow, deep breaths, allowing your mind to quiet.

2. **Create your scene.** Begin to visualize yourself sitting on a peaceful beach. Feel the warmth of the sun on your skin, the gentle breeze on your face, and the sand supporting you beneath your body. In front of you, the ocean stretches wide and endless, its surface rising and falling in a steady rhythm. This is a safe space; calm, open, and filled with the sound of waves that match the pace of your breath.
3. **Connect your breath to the waves.** As you inhale, imagine the waves rolling toward you, each one carrying an emotion or thought that has surfaced within you. Allow yourself to notice what arises; there's no need to label or resist it. Just breathe in and witness what the water brings.
4. **Release with the exhale.** As you exhale, visualize the waves retreating back into the ocean, carrying away your distressing emotions, worries, or heaviness. Watch them dissolve into the vast water, leaving the shore smooth and quiet again. With each exhale, feel a little lighter, a little clearer.
5. **Flow with the rhythm.** Continue this visualization for several minutes, letting your breath and the movement of the waves merge into one steady rhythm. Allow emotions to come and go freely, trusting that each one will return to the ocean when it's ready. There's nothing to fix, only to feel and release.
6. **Return to presence.** When you feel complete, take a few final deep breaths and slowly bring your awareness back to your body. Feel the surface beneath you, the air around you, and the calm that now rests inside. Carry with you the sense that, like the ocean, your emotions have tides, they rise, they fall, and they always return to stillness.

Heartfelt Gratitude List

Anchor yourself in the present through the practice of gratitude. This technique shifts your focus away from uncomfortable emotions by nurturing a sense of appreciation for the positives in your life.

Instructions

1. **Prepare your space.** Find a quiet, comfortable place where you can sit without interruptions. Take a few slow breaths to

center yourself and gently shift your focus inward, leaving behind the distractions of your day.

2. **Set your intention.** For about 10 minutes, let your thoughts flow freely. Reflect on at least 10 things you feel grateful for. These can be big or small: people, experiences, moments of beauty, or even simple comforts like a warm meal or a good night's sleep.
3. **Reflect as you note your observations.** As you note each item, pause for a moment to reflect on why you're grateful for it. Think about how it enriches your life or how it makes you feel supported, loved, or at peace. Let yourself experience the emotion of gratitude fully.
4. **Let the feeling expand.** With each reflection, notice how your body responds, perhaps a softening in your chest, a deeper breath, or a sense of warmth spreading through you. Allow each positive memory or feeling to fill you with a quiet contentment, grounding you in the present moment.
5. **Review and integrate.** As you finish, notice how abundance shows up in both ordinary and extraordinary ways. Close your eyes and take a deep breath, letting gratitude wash through you like a steady, grounding current. Carry this feeling with you as a reminder that even in difficult times, moments of goodness are always within reach.

Key Takeaways

- This chapter highlighted how tuning in to subtle physical sensations can reveal deeper emotional truths and offer a pathway to healing. By cultivating your internal observation skills, you unlock the potential for self-awareness, allowing you to address stressors and emotional struggles more effectively.
- This journey of self-discovery is accessible to anyone willing to embrace it with curiosity and compassion. With consistent practice, interoceptive awareness becomes a nurturing ritual that enhances your emotional resilience and strengthens your relationship with yourself. You'll learn to listen to your body's messages, gaining clarity and insight into the connection between your physical sensations and emotions.

Traveling the path of somatic body awareness offers lifelong benefits that reach far beyond the physical. As you deepen this connection with yourself, you cultivate greater emotional resilience and a sense of inner balance, qualities that support well-being in today's fast-paced world.

In the next chapter, I'll share some of the somatic practices that supported me most in my own healing journey. These exercises are designed to help you gently manage PTSD symptoms, release stored tension, and rebuild a sense of safety and trust within your body.

04.

Somatic Exercises for Coping With PTSD

You can't stop the waves,
but you can learn to surf. –Jon Kabat-Zinn

"

Post-Traumatic Stress Disorder (PTSD) is a condition that can develop after experiencing or witnessing a distressing or life-threatening event. It affects both the mind and body, often leading to symptoms such as intrusive memories, hypervigilance, anxiety, or a feeling of disconnection from oneself and others. What's important to understand is that trauma isn't stored only in thoughts; it also lives in the body, influencing how we breathe, move, and respond to stress.

Coping with PTSD through somatic exercises means learning to gently reconnect with your body and rebuild a sense of safety from within. These practices use awareness of movement, breath, and physical sensations to calm the nervous system and bring you back to the present moment. They can be powerful tools for finding steadiness when emotions feel intense or overwhelming.

In my own experience, reconnecting with the body in this way created a bridge between survival and healing. Somatic work reminded me that even after trauma, the body holds an incredible capacity for resilience and recovery. The techniques in this chapter are designed to help you discover this same sense of stability and empowerment in your own healing process.

Breathwork Techniques for Calming the Nervous System

Even though breathing happens automatically, intentional breathwork can be a powerful tool for healing. When you bring awareness to your breath, you do more than calm your mind; you engage your body's natural ability to regulate and restore balance.

Deep breathing, in particular, has a profound effect on your physiology. It stimulates the vagus nerve, which activates the parasympathetic nervous system, the part responsible for bringing your body into a relaxed "rest and digest" state.

Under stress, the breath becomes shallow and fast, typically between 12 to 20 breaths per minute. But when you consciously slow your breath to about 5 to 7 breaths per minute, something incredible happens. Your heart rate begins to lower, your blood pressure stabilizes, and your brain receives the signal that you are safe. This gentle shift is your body's invitation to relax and release the tension it's been holding.

But there's more happening beneath the surface. While most of us are taught to focus on oxygen intake, carbon dioxide is just as vital. Shallow breathing often causes levels to drop too low, which can lead to dizziness, anxiety, and reduced oxygen delivery to your brain and muscles. Deep, rhythmic breathing restores the balance between oxygen and carbon dioxide, optimizing both cellular function and emotional regulation. You're not just breathing to survive; you're breathing to *heal.*

By incorporating breathwork into your daily routine, especially during triggering or dysregulated moments, you can regulate your emotional responses, access clarity, and develop a deeper sense of internal safety. In the sections ahead, we'll explore simple yet powerful techniques that support nervous system regulation and emotional resilience, helping you shift from panic to presence, one conscious breath at a time.

Deep Belly Breathing

Deep belly breathing invites you to breathe deeply through your nose, allowing air to fill your abdomen, and slowly releasing your breath through your mouth. By honing in on these sensations, anxiety can often be quelled, providing a momentary respite from intrusive thoughts and overwhelming emotions.

Here are guidelines for practicing deep belly breathing:

1. Choose a quiet area in your home or office where you won't be disturbed. Sit in a comfortable chair or lie down on your back with your knees bent and feet flat on the floor.
2. Close your eyes if you feel comfortable doing so. Take a moment to relax your shoulders, neck, and jaw. Allow your body to settle into a calm state.
3. Rest one hand on your chest and the other on your abdomen. This will help you monitor your breathing and ensure you are using your diaphragm.
4. Inhale slowly through your nose for a count of four. As you breathe in, feel your abdomen rise as your diaphragm expands. Your chest should remain relatively still.
5. Hold your breath for a count of two. This brief pause allows your body to fully absorb oxygen.
6. Exhale slowly and completely through your mouth for a count of six. Feel your abdomen fall as you release the air.
7. Continue this cycle of deep breathing for 5–10 minutes. Focus on the rhythm of your breath, allowing your mind to clear.
8. Consider incorporating a mantra or positive affirmation during your practice to enhance mindfulness. Examples include *"I am calm"* or *"I am in control."*
9. Experiment with different positions such as standing, sitting cross-legged on the floor, or even doing diaphragmatic breathing during a walk. This makes the practice adaptable and personal.

Box Breathing

Transitioning to box breathing, this method provides structure through its balanced inhalation and exhalation processes. This rhythmic pattern builds mindfulness and serves to harmonize your body's responses. In moments of heightened stress, engaging in this exercise can stabilize your emotional state and enhance your concentration.

Here are simple steps to practice box breathing:

1. Choose a quiet and comfortable spot at home or in the office where you can sit or stand without distractions.
2. Decide how long you want to practice box breathing. You can start with a few minutes. Use a timer app on your phone that offers soothing sounds or visuals during your session to make it more enjoyable.
3. Sit or stand with your back straight and shoulders relaxed. It's important to find a position that feels most natural and comfortable for you, whether that's in a chair, on the floor, or standing.
4. Gently close your eyes to minimize distractions. If you're uncomfortable closing your eyes, focus on a specific point in front of you instead. You can also use a calming eye mask to enhance relaxation.
5. Breathe in slowly through your nose for a count of four (4 seconds). After inhaling, hold your breath for another count of four (4 seconds). Breathe out through your mouth for a count of four (4 seconds). After exhaling, pause for a count of four (4 seconds).
6. Continue the cycle of inhaling, holding, exhaling, and pausing for several minutes. Feel free to adjust the counts to suit your comfort level, gradually increasing the duration as you become more accustomed to the exercise. After finishing, take a moment to reflect on how you feel.

Alternate Nostril Breathing

For those seeking to balance their energy flow, alternate nostril breathing offers a unique approach. By consciously alternating the nostril used for inhalation and exhalation, a synchronization of your brain's hemispheres is achieved (Singh et al., n.d.). This balance aids in deepening clarity and cultivating a state of inner calm.

Here are instructions you can follow to practice alternate nostril breathing:

1. Sit cross-legged on the floor or in a chair with your feet flat on the ground. Ensure your back is straight and your shoulders are relaxed.
2. Bring your right hand up toward your face, allowing your thumb to rest on your right nostril and your ring finger to rest on your left nostril. Your index and middle fingers can gently rest on your forehead or be curled into your palm.
3. Use your thumb to gently press against your right nostril, closing it off fully.
4. Take a deep, slow breath in through your left nostril, filling your lungs completely.
5. After inhaling, use your ring finger to close your left nostril, releasing your thumb from your right nostril.
6. Breathe out completely through your right nostril, emptying your lungs.
7. After fully exhaling, lift your thumb off your right nostril and inhale deeply and slowly through it.
8. Press your thumb back against your right nostril after inhaling.
9. Release your ring finger from your left nostril and exhale slowly and fully through your left nostril.
10. This completes one round of alternate nostril breathing. Repeat this process for several rounds, focusing on your breath and finding a rhythm that feels comfortable for you.

11. After a few rounds, take a moment to breathe normally and notice how you feel, both physically and mentally. When you're ready, gently open your eyes and bring your awareness back to the room.

Humming Breath

In addition to these practices, humming breath introduces another layer of engagement. This technique involves taking a deep inhalation and producing a gentle humming sound during exhalation. The vibrational quality of the hum creates a soothing effect that resonates through your body. These vibrations have the potential to ground you in your physical presence, building a deeper connection with your emotions. By concentrating on the sensation of the hum, you may find yourself more emotionally attuned, facilitating a pathway to internal peace.

Consider the following steps when practicing the humming breath:

1. Sit in a cross-legged position on the floor or in a chair with your back straight and shoulders relaxed. Rest your hands on your knees or in your lap.
2. Gently close your eyes to minimize distractions and help focus on your breath and sounds.
3. Inhale deeply through your nose, filling your lungs and expanding your diaphragm. Hold your breath for a moment.
4. As you exhale slowly through your mouth, produce a gentle humming sound. Aim for a pitch that feels comfortable, allowing the vibration to resonate in your body.
5. Pay attention to the vibrations created by the hum. Notice how they travel through your throat, chest, and head. Allow this awareness to deepen your relaxation.
6. Inhale again deeply and hum on your exhale. Practice this for 5–10 minutes, maintaining a steady rhythm. Let your humming flow naturally.
7. After a few minutes, try changing the pitch of your hum, exploring lower or higher frequencies to see how it affects your experience.

8. As you hum, visualize the soundwaves radiating from your body, spreading calm and relaxation throughout your space.
9. When you feel ready, gradually reduce the volume of your humming and take a few deep breaths before slowly opening your eyes. Take a moment to notice how you feel.
10. Spend a minute reflecting on your experience, journaling about any insights or feelings that arose during the practice.

Like most holistic practices, breathwork becomes more effective with consistency. The more often you practice, the more naturally your body learns to find calm and balance. I've found it helpful to experiment with different breathing techniques to see which ones feel most supportive; some feel grounding, while others are energizing. There's no single right way to breathe intentionally; what matters is finding what fits you. The beauty of breathwork is its flexibility; you can adapt it to your mood, your schedule, and where you are on your healing journey.

Visualization Exercises for Emotional Release

In your healing journey, visualization can be a powerful ally for processing emotions and releasing trauma. These guided imagery practices invite you to connect with your inner world in a safe, intentional way, allowing buried feelings and memories to surface gently, without overwhelm. Through visualization, you can reshape how your body and mind relate to past experiences, creating space for calm and renewed perspective.

In the following pages, you'll find a few simple yet powerful visualization techniques designed to support emotional release and help you reconnect with a sense of inner peace.

Safe Space Visualization

Safe space visualization involves creating a mental refuge where you can safely explore and handle difficult emotions without becoming overwhelmed. The aim is to create a mental sanctuary where you can slowly and gently confront difficult emotions and experiences, much like easing into a warm bath after a long day. This practice does not rush the healing process but instead provides a stable foundation from which to courageously face the weight of traumatic memories.

Follow this visualization script to practice safe space visualization:

1. Begin by finding a comfortable position, either seated or lying down, and gently close your eyes. Take a deep breath in through your nose, allowing your belly to expand, and then exhale slowly through your mouth. With each breath, let go of any tension or worries, feeling your body sink deeper into relaxation.

2. Visualize a place where you feel completely safe and secure. This can be a real location, like a cozy room in your home, or an imaginary space, such as a magical forest or a serene beach. Picture the details vividly: the colors, the textures, and the sounds.

3. As you envision your safe space, engage all of your senses. What do you see? Are there vibrant colors or soft lighting? What do you hear? Perhaps the gentle rustle of leaves or the soothing sound of waves? What do you smell? Take in the fragrance of flowers, fresh air, or warm wood. How does the ground feel beneath you? Is it soft grass or warm sand? Allow these sensory details to immerse you further into your safe space.

4. Introduce elements that bring you comfort into your visualization. Picture soft cushions or blankets where you can rest. Imagine a warm cup of tea or your favorite book nearby. Visualize any objects that provide you with a sense of security, like a cherished stuffed animal or a protective crystal.

5. Expand your awareness of the surroundings in your safe space. Are there trees gently swaying in the breeze? Is there a clear blue sky above you? Focus on the peacefulness of the environment, making it as vibrant and life-like as possible.

6. Once you're comfortable, envision a gentle protective barrier surrounding your safe space. This could be a warm light, a soft cloud, or a sparkling bubble that shields you from negativity, stress, or any outside disturbances. Visualize this barrier glowing softly, ensuring you feel completely at ease.

7. As you settle into your safe space, invite positive energies and feelings to surround you. Imagine a warm, glowing light filling your heart, bringing joy, calmness, and serenity. Let this energy gradually expand to fill every part of your safe space.
8. Spend a few moments in this safe space, allowing your mind and body to relax fully. Remind yourself that you can return to this place anytime you need to feel secure and at peace. When you're ready, slowly start to return to the present, taking with you a sense of calm and safety.
9. Begin to wiggle your fingers and toes, bringing awareness back to your body. Open your eyes gently when you feel ready, taking a moment to notice how you feel. Carry the peace of your safe space with you into your day.

Releasing Visualization

Releasing visualization involves using vivid imagery to let go of pent-up emotions, often symbolized through interactions with nature, like envisioning your worries as leaves floating down a river. This imagery helps reinforce the idea that emotions are temporary, transient, and ultimately manageable. For instance, you might picture anger, sadness, or fear as colorful balloons that you release into the sky, watching them disappear among the clouds. This particular visualization empowers you to see your emotions as manageable entities rather than overwhelming forces, building a sense of control and liberation.

Follow the script below to carry out the releasing visualization:

1. Sit or stand with your back straight and shoulders relaxed. It's important to find a position that feels most natural and comfortable for you, whether that's in a chair, on the floor, or standing.
2. Visualize roots extending from the base of your spine or your feet, growing deep into the earth. Imagine these roots anchoring you, connecting you to the stability of the ground below, providing you with a sense of security and calm.
3. Focus on your breathing. Inhale slowly through your nose, allowing your abdomen to expand fully. Hold that breath for

a moment, then exhale gently through your mouth, releasing any tension. Continue this deep breathing, imagining each inhalation filling you with light and clarity and each exhalation releasing negativity and stress.

4. Picture a small, swirling ball of light at the center of your chest, representing your worries, fears, or negative emotions. With each breath, visualize this ball growing brighter and lighter, fueled by your intention to release these burdens.
5. As you exhale, imagine the ball of light floating out of your chest and expanding into a radiant, glowing orb. With each breath out, see it growing larger and more luminous, transforming all the negativity into beautiful, soothing energy.
6. With your next inhale, visualize the orb gently rising above you, carrying away all that no longer serves you. See it drifting up into the sky, becoming lighter and brighter as it ascends. Feel a sense of relief as you let go of every worry and fear, trusting the universe to take care of you.
7. As the orb disappears into the vastness, bring your focus back to your breath. Imagine the space within you now filled with warmth, love, and light. Visualize this energy spreading throughout your body, filling every cell with positivity and peace.
8. Gradually bring your awareness back to your surroundings. Wiggle your fingers and toes, reconnecting with your body. When you're ready, open your eyes gently. Take a moment to notice how you feel, embracing the lightness that comes from releasing what no longer serves you.

Future Self Visualization

Future self visualization shifts your focus toward an empowering vision of yourself. It encourages you to imagine who you might become, free from the constraints of past trauma. This future self acts as a guide and a beacon of hope, offering motivation and purpose in your healing journey. Envisioning such a future can rekindle aspirations once lost to trauma's grip, serving as a compelling reminder of the potential for transformation.

Here is a script to practice future self visualization:

1. Begin by finding a comfortable position, either seated or lying down, and gently close your eyes. Take a deep breath in through your nose, allowing your belly to expand, and then exhale slowly through your mouth. With each breath, let go of any tension or worries, feeling your body sink deeper into relaxation.
2. Visualize a beautiful door in front of you, representing the gateway to your future self. Take a moment to appreciate the design of the door—its color, texture, and any unique features. Feel the anticipation building as you prepare to open it.
3. Slowly reach for the doorknob and feel the cool metal against your palm. As you turn the knob, notice the gentle creaking of the door as it swings open, revealing a radiant light on the other side.
4. Step through the door into a vibrant, expansive landscape that represents your future. Observe the details of this place—the colors, sounds, and scents that surround you. Allow yourself to feel the energy of this future environment.
5. In the distance, you spot your future self standing confidently. Take a moment to examine this version of yourself. What are they wearing? What expressions are on their face? Notice the posture and the aura of confidence radiating from them.
6. As you approach your future self, feel the warmth and positivity flowing from them. Engage in a conversation; ask them what achievements and experiences have led them to this moment. Listen closely to their insights and advice.
7. Envision yourself adopting their qualities—confidence, wisdom, and strength. Imagine integrating these traits into your current self, feeling the transformation taking place within you.
8. Now, reflect on the specific goals and aspirations that your future self has accomplished. Visualize the steps and decisions that led to these successes, creating a detailed road map in your mind.
9. Take a moment to express gratitude to your future self for the guidance and inspiration they've provided. Feel the connection between the two of you strengthen as you appreciate this moment of clarity.

10. To conclude the visualization, slowly step back through the door, bringing with you feelings of hope, empowerment, and clarity. Close the door gently behind you, knowing you can return to this space whenever you need.

Emotional Color Visualization

Color plays a pivotal role in visualization practices, helping you creatively explore complex emotions. Emotional color visualization harnesses the psychological impact colors possess, enabling you to express feelings artistically. Think of how different colors evoke various moods: a deep blue might represent calm, while a fiery red could symbolize anger. By assigning colors to emotions, you can paint mental pictures that help you understand and process these feelings more deeply.

The script below will help you practice emotional color visualization:

1. Begin by finding a comfortable position, closing your eyes, and taking a deep breath.
2. Think of a specific emotion you want to visualize. It could be joy, sadness, anger, or peace. Identify the color that you associate most strongly with this emotion.
3. Picture your chosen color in your mind. Imagine it as a soft, glowing ball of light. Visualize this colored light beginning to fill the space around you, illuminating everything it touches.
4. As you visualize this color, allow yourself to fully experience the emotion associated with it. What does it feel like in your body? Where do you feel it the strongest? Let this emotion wash over you.
5. Now, picture this colored light entering your body. Imagine it entering through the top of your head and slowly spreading throughout your entire being. Feel the warmth and vibrancy of the color filling every part of you.
6. As the color flows through you, allow it to grow stronger. Imagine it pulsating with energy, and allow this energy to enhance the feelings associated with the color. Let it uplift you or provide the comfort you need.

7. See yourself interacting with this color, such as painting a canvas with it or enveloping your loved ones with its light. Imagine this interaction amplifying your emotional experience.
8. Think of shapes, symbols, or scenes that represent your emotion. For example, if you are visualizing joy, you might picture bright, vibrant flowers or the sun shining. If you are feeling sadness, you might visualize rain or a calm ocean.
9. After you've immersed yourself in this emotional color visualization, slowly begin to bring your attention back to the present moment. Gradually allow the colors to fade but keep the emotional resonance with you.

Movement Practices for Releasing Trauma

The connection between your body and mind runs deep, and understanding it can change the way you approach healing. Trauma isn't only something we think about; it's something we *carry*. It can live in our muscles, tissues, and posture, showing up as tension, fatigue, or a sense of disconnection from ourselves.

When I began to move with awareness, through stretching, gentle yoga, and even simple walking, I started to feel emotions I hadn't realized were still living in my body. Movement became more than exercise; it became a way to release what words couldn't reach.

In the pages ahead, you'll explore a variety of movement-based practices that can help you gently release stored emotion, restore energy flow, and reconnect with your body. Each one offers an opportunity to move toward wholeness, presence, and empowerment, one mindful motion at a time.

Shaking or Vibrating Exercise

Shaking or vibrating are spontaneous body movements aimed at releasing tension and discharging stress. The beauty of this exercise lies in its simplicity—you can do it without prior training or equipment.

Music can further enhance the experience, allowing you to feel more connected and engaged with your movements. By selecting music that resonates emotionally, you can travel deeper into your unconscious mind, shaking loose any buried emotions just below the surface. This method serves as both a liberating and grounding practice, encouraging you to reconnect with your body and the present moment.

Here are guidelines for practicing shaking or vibrating for trauma release:

1. Before starting, take a moment to connect with your body and the ground. Stand or sit with your feet firmly planted, close your eyes, and take deep breaths, allowing your belly to expand. Feel the support of the ground beneath you.
2. Take a moment to reflect on what you hope to achieve through this practice. Whether it's to release tension, stress, or trauma, stating your intention can help focus your energy.
3. Begin by gently shaking your hands, wrists, and arms at your sides. Allow the motion to be organic and free, gradually increasing the intensity. Pay close attention to how your body responds.
4. Sync your shaking with deep breathing. Inhale deeply through your nose, allowing your abdomen to expand, then exhale through your mouth, releasing all tension. Let your breath guide the rhythm of your movements.
5. As you become more comfortable, expand your shaking to involve your legs and torso. Let your entire body participate—allow your knees to bend, your hips to move, and feel your feet lift slightly off the ground if it feels right.
6. Allow sounds to accompany your shaking if you feel called to do so. This can include humming, chanting, or even vocalizing emotions. Letting out sound can enhance the release process and help express what is within.
7. Experiment with varying the speed and intensity of your shaking. Alternate between fast, energetic movements and slower, more controlled shakes. Notice how these changes affect your emotional state.
8. Throughout the practice, maintain a connection with your body and emotions. If certain feelings or memories arise, acknowledge them without judgment, allowing yourself to feel them as they come.

9. After engaging in shaking for a period of time (10–20 minutes), gradually slow down your movements. Transition into stillness, taking deep breaths and sitting or lying down to reflect on the experience.

Dance Movement Therapy

Dance Movement Therapy (DMT) is a form of creative art psychotherapy that uses improvised dance to express deep thoughts and feelings without words, serving as a dynamic tool for emotional processing. Unlike structured dance forms, it emphasizes spontaneity and creative expression, letting you explore your inner world through movement. Through DMT, you gain heightened emotional awareness, enhancing your self-awareness and empathy toward others. By engaging in this therapeutic form, you often find you can break away from cognitive restraints and experience an authentic release—a freedom drawn from dance's innate ability to transcend verbal limitations.

Below is a simple and fun dance movement exercise to expose you to this creative technique:

1. Begin with gentle stretching of your arms, legs, and torso to prepare your body. Spend about 5 minutes loosening up.
2. Stand with your feet hip-width apart. Shift your weight to your right foot and lift your left foot slightly off the ground, then switch and repeat for eight counts.
3. While performing the basic step, add arm movements. Reach your arms up overhead as you shift your weight to the right, then bring your arms down as you switch to the left, creating a fluid motion.
4. After eight counts of the basic step with arm movements, incorporate a gentle twist in your torso. As you move to the right, turn your torso to face the right, then switch to face the left on the next step.
5. Combine the basic steps, arm movements, and rotation. Do this for sixteen counts, focusing on making smooth transitions between each element.

6. For the last two minutes, let loose! Play your favorite song and improvise your own movements, incorporating what you've practiced. Allow your body to move freely and express yourself.
7. Finish with deep breaths and gentle stretches to relax your muscles.

Gentle Yoga

Gentle yoga became one of the practices that helped me reconnect with my body after trauma. The slow, mindful movements and stretches created a safe space to breathe, release tension, and simply be in my body again.

This approach encourages you to move with awareness and compassion, responding to your body's cues and limits as they arise. Through steady, intentional practice, these movements help release the stress and emotion held in your muscles, creating a deeper sense of ease, balance, and trust within yourself.

Unlike intense yoga styles focused on achieving difficult postures, gentle yoga is about honoring your body and embracing comfort in stillness and flow. It provides a safe space to explore physical boundaries while cultivating mindfulness and patience. You learn the value of breathing deeply in sync with each pose, building an environment of calm and introspection. As you unearth stored tensions, there's a noticeable shift in your body's energy flow, leading to increased physical and mental clarity.

Here are five easy-to-follow, gentle yoga poses that you can practice at home. If you enjoy them, browse for more poses on sites like YouTube, where you can find demonstrations, or take a class at a nearby yoga studio.

Downward-Facing Dog (*Adho Mukha Svanasana*)

This pose resembles an inverted V shape and is excellent for stretching the entire body. It helps to strengthen the arms, legs, and back while also improving circulation and relieving stress.

Instructions:

1. **Begin on all fours.** Come to your hands and knees with your wrists aligned under your shoulders and your knees beneath your hips. Spread your fingers wide, pressing your palms evenly into the mat to create a stable base.
2. **Lift your hips.** Tuck your toes under and, on an exhale, gently lift your knees away from the floor. Slowly straighten your legs as you raise your hips toward the ceiling, forming an inverted "V" shape.
3. **Adjust your position.** Keep your hands shoulder-width apart and your feet about hip-width apart. Let your head and neck relax, allowing your gaze to rest softly between your feet.
4. **Find your alignment.** Press your heels toward the ground—it's okay if they don't touch. Focus on lengthening through your spine rather than forcing the stretch. Keep a gentle bend in your knees if needed to avoid strain in your lower back.
5. **Breathe and settle.** Take several slow, steady breaths here. Feel the stretch along the back of your legs, through your shoulders, and down your spine. With each exhale, imagine releasing tension from your body and softening into the pose.
6. **Return to rest.** When you're ready to come out of the pose, lower your knees gently back to the mat and rest in Child's Pose or on your forearms for a few breaths. Notice the sensations in your body, the warmth, energy, or lightness that may arise.

Child's Pose (*Balasana*)

The child's pose is a common resting position that promotes relaxation and gentle stretching. It calms the mind and relieves tension in the back and shoulders, too.

Instructions:

1. **Begin on your mat**. Start in a kneeling position with your big toes touching and your knees either together or slightly apart—whichever feels more comfortable for your hips.

2. **Fold forward.** Sit back on your heels and slowly walk your hands forward, lowering your chest toward the ground. Allow your forehead to rest softly on the mat, a cushion, or stacked hands if needed for support.
3. **Settle and adjust.** Extend your arms fully in front of you for an active stretch through the spine and shoulders or keep them alongside your body with palms facing up for a more restorative variation. Let your elbows and shoulders relax completely.
4. **Breathe with awareness.** Begin to take slow, deep breaths in through your nose and out through your mouth. With each inhale, feel your back expanding gently; with each exhale, allow your body to release a little more tension into the ground.
5. **Stay and observe.** Remain here for several breaths or as long as it feels supportive. Notice the sensation of safety and stillness in this position. When you're ready, press your palms into the mat and slowly roll up to a seated position, carrying that sense of calm with you.

Cat–Cow Stretch (*Marjaryasana–Bitilasana*)

This stretch is a dynamic yoga pose that transitions fluidly between the cat and cow positions. This flowing sequence promotes flexibility of the spine, enhances mobility, and eases tension in the back, creating a calming rhythm for both body and mind.

Instructions:

1. **Find your starting position.** Begin on your hands and knees in a tabletop position. Align your wrists directly under your shoulders and your knees beneath your hips. Spread your fingers wide and press your palms evenly into the mat to create a stable foundation.
2. **Move into Cow Pose.** As you inhale, slowly arch your back. Drop your belly toward the floor while lifting your chest and tailbone toward the ceiling. Draw your shoulders away from your ears and let your gaze lift slightly forward or upward. Feel a gentle stretch across the front of your torso and spine.

3. **Transition to Cat Pose.** On your exhale, reverse the movement. Round your spine toward the ceiling, tucking your chin toward your chest and drawing your navel in toward your spine. Allow your head and neck to relax as you feel a stretch through your upper and middle back.

4. **Create a steady rhythm.** Continue flowing between Cat and Cow for several slow, intentional breaths—inhale to arch, exhale to round. Let the motion follow your breathing, allowing each movement to feel smooth and natural. Notice how your spine begins to loosen and your body feels more fluid with each cycle.

5. **Finish mindfully.** When you're ready to close the sequence, return to a neutral tabletop position. Take a moment to notice the sensations in your back and shoulders and feel the subtle warmth and calm energy this movement creates.

Seated Forward Bend (*Paschimottanasana*)

Paschimottanasana, or Seated Forward Bend, is a fundamental seated yoga pose that provides a deep stretch to the entire back and hamstrings. This pose is not only beneficial for physical flexibility but also encourages a sense of calmness and introspection by promoting relaxation and focus.

Instructions:

1. **Find your starting position.** Sit on your mat with your legs extended straight in front of you. Flex your feet gently so your toes point upward and your heels rest on the mat. If your hamstrings feel tight, you can place a folded blanket or cushion under your hips to support a tall spine.

2. **Lengthen your posture.** Inhale deeply and sit up straight, lengthening through the crown of your head. Imagine creating space between each vertebra. Roll your shoulders back and let your arms rest at your sides.

3. **Hinge forward from your hips.** As you exhale, begin to fold forward from the hips rather than rounding your back. Keep your spine long as you reach your hands toward your feet,

ankles, or shins, wherever they naturally land. The goal is to move with awareness, not to push or force the stretch.

4. **Soften into the pose.** Once you find your edge, allow your head and neck to relax, and take a few slow, steady breaths. With each inhale, imagine lengthening your spine just a little more; with each exhale, allow your body to release deeper into the stretch.
5. **Stay and breathe.** Hold the pose for several breaths or up to a minute, letting your body gradually open. Notice any sensations of release through your back and legs, and allow a feeling of calm to settle in.
6. **Return gently.** To come out of the pose, engage your core and slowly roll your spine upward, one vertebra at a time, until you're sitting tall again. Take a moment to observe how your body feels, perhaps more open, grounded, and at ease.

Corpse Pose (*Savasana*)

Savasana, known as the ultimate relaxation pose, is a cornerstone of yoga practice that allows the body to fully absorb the benefits of previous asanas. This posture serves as a bridge between active practice and mindful stillness, providing an opportunity to rejuvenate your body and mind.

Instructions:

1. **Find your position.** Lie flat on your back with your legs extended comfortably. Let your feet fall open naturally, allowing the hips to release. If your lower back feels tense, you can place a rolled blanket or bolster under your knees for support.
2. **Rest your arms and settle in.** Allow your arms to rest alongside your body, palms facing upward in a gesture of openness. Soften your shoulders away from your ears and release any tightness in your hands or fingers.
3. **Close your eyes and arrive.** Gently close your eyes and bring your attention inward. Begin to notice your breath

without trying to change it, just observe its natural rhythm as it flows in and out.

4. **Release and relax.** With each exhale, invite your body to sink a little deeper into the surface beneath you. Imagine your weight melting downward as tension leaves your jaw, neck, chest, and abdomen. Allow your entire body to feel supported and safe.

5. **Rest in stillness.** Remain here for several minutes, letting your breath become smooth and effortless. If your mind begins to wander, gently bring your focus back to the rise and fall of your breath or the sensations of your body resting.

6. **Return gently.** When you're ready to come out of the pose, start by deepening your breath. Wiggle your fingers and toes to reawaken your body. Slowly roll to one side into a fetal position, pausing for a moment before pressing yourself up to a seated position. Take a final breath of gratitude for the stillness and release you've created.

Through these movement-based practices, you may begin to discover simple yet powerful ways to manage PTSD symptoms in your daily life. Each exercise helps you reconnect with your body, reminding you that healing unfolds through both physical and emotional awareness. Recovery is not something that happens only in the mind or only in the body; it lives in the dialogue between the two. By nurturing this connection, you open the door to greater balance, resilience, and a deeper sense of personal empowerment.

Key Takeaways

- Breathwork, visualization, and movement practices offer tangible methods for calming your nervous system, reducing anxiety, and enhancing focus.
- The simplicity and accessibility of these exercises make them invaluable tools that seamlessly integrate into your daily life, promoting resilience even in stressful environments.
- These exercises provide more than just temporary relief; they empower you by offering control over your physiological responses and emotions.

By regularly practicing these techniques, you can gradually ease the intensity of PTSD symptoms and build a stronger sense of peace, confidence, and self-awareness. Each step you take through somatic movement and breathwork supports your ongoing growth, helping you create a stable foundation for healing and resilience.

In the next chapter, we'll broaden our view to explore how somatic therapy is understood and practiced across different cultures. By examining these diverse perspectives, you'll gain a deeper appreciation for the universal wisdom behind body-based healing and the many ways it continues to evolve around the world.

05.

Cultural Perspectives on Somatic Therapy

Each of us has a unique part to play in the healing of the world. –Marianne Williamson

“

The way we experience healing is deeply influenced by the culture we come from. Our beliefs, traditions, and community stories shape how we understand the body, what we consider "healing," and how we connect to our own inner wisdom. Around the world, somatic practices may look different on the surface, whether it's yoga in India, qigong in China, Indigenous ceremonies, or Western bodywork, but they all share a common understanding: that healing involves the whole person, not just the body's symptoms.

When we look through a cultural lens, we begin to see how our backgrounds, our spirituality, family systems, and collective histories inform the way we process pain and seek balance. Some cultures have always viewed the body as sacred, a vessel of energy and intuition, while others are only beginning to rediscover this wisdom. By exploring these perspectives, we can learn new ways to approach healing and deepen our appreciation for how universal the connection between body and spirit truly is.

Cultural Variations in Body-Mind Healing Practices

In many cultures, healing is understood as something much deeper than the treatment of physical symptoms. Within Indigenous traditions, especially, healing is woven into the fabric of community life. It's not just a personal process; it's a shared experience that connects people to their ancestors, their stories, and the natural world. Ceremonies, rituals, and storytelling are often central to this approach, helping individuals restore harmony within themselves and within the collective.

For example, among some Native American tribes, the use of sweat lodges represents much more than physical purification. The experience is meant to cleanse both body and spirit, helping participants release emotional burdens and reconnect with a sense of inner clarity. The ceremony takes place within a sacred, communal space where people pray, sing, and reflect together, reinforcing bonds of community and cultural identity (Zermeño & Laster Pirtle, 2021).

Similarly, the Māori of New Zealand incorporate their language, customs, and ancestral wisdom into healing practices, showing how deeply culture influences well-being. In these traditions, storytelling, ritual, and community connection are just as essential as the therapeutic process itself. Healing is understood as something that involves the whole person, mind, body, and spirit, and it unfolds in relationship with the land, the ancestors, and the community.

In contrast, many Eastern traditions, particularly those found across parts of Asia, focus on emotional balance and inner awareness as the foundation for well-being. Mindfulness and movement practices like yoga and tai chi are not seen as just forms of exercise, but as ways to bring the body and mind into harmony. These traditions invite practitioners to slow down, breathe with intention, and cultivate presence, creating a sense of calm, balance, and emotional stability that supports overall health.

Mindfulness, a cornerstone of many Eastern philosophies, teaches the value of being fully present. By bringing attention to the here and now, it helps quiet the mind, ease anxiety, and reduce stress, offering a very different rhythm of healing compared to the often future-focused, problem-solving approach found in Western therapy.

Movement practices like Qi Gong integrate gentle, intentional motion with deep breathing and meditation, illustrating how emotional calm and physical flow are closely connected. Within these traditions, health is seen as a state of harmony where the mind and body continuously influence and support each other.

Community support also plays a central role in many Indigenous healing traditions around the world. These approaches recognize that healing doesn't happen in isolation; it's strengthened through connection and shared experience.

In many African traditions, for instance, traditional healers may invite a person's family or wider community to participate in the process, creating a circle of emotional, spiritual, and sometimes even financial support. This collective involvement reminds us that empowerment often grows through belonging, and that community itself can be one of the most powerful medicines.

By including community participation as part of the healing process, many cultures emphasize that isolation works against well-being. Healing, in these contexts, grows through shared experience and collective care. When people feel seen, supported, and connected, it strengthens the environment in which recovery can take place. This view contrasts with many Western models that often prioritize privacy and individual responsibility in therapy, revealing how differently cultures can define what it means to be well.

Successfully integrating somatic therapies across different cultures requires awareness, respect, and flexibility. Every healing approach carries its own cultural wisdom, and when we bring somatic practices into diverse settings, it's important to adapt them with care.

By exploring and honoring various healing traditions, you can shape these techniques to fit your own values and cultural background. This kind of personal alignment not only deepens connection to the practice but also makes the therapeutic process more meaningful and effective.

Different Somatic Practices From Across the Globe

Cultural background greatly influences how people approach healing and body awareness. Around the world, different communities have developed somatic practices that reflect their philosophies, values, and ways of understanding the connection between mind, body, and spirit. Each tradition carries its own rhythm and wisdom, offering unique insights into how movement, breath, and presence can restore balance and vitality.

I encourage you to explore some of these practices; try them at home, learn about their origins, or simply reflect on which ones resonate most with you. Each holds valuable lessons about how healing deepens when it honors both the individual and the culture it comes from.

Qigong (China)

Qigong is a centuries-old practice that embodies a blend of slow movements and meditation, rooted deeply in Chinese philosophy. The essence of Qigong is to cultivate "Qi," or life energy, through deliberate, slow movements and focused breathwork (Jahnke et al., 2010). By incorporating techniques that enhance concentration and mindful awareness, Qigong facilitates healing both physically and emotionally, providing a pathway to inner peace and self-awareness. Its meditative nature allows you to access a state of calm, essential for managing stress and promoting holistic well-being.

Here is a beginner-friendly Qigong exercise that you can practice at home:

1. Stand with your feet shoulder-width apart, knees slightly bent, arms relaxed by your sides, and hands open. This is known as the "Wu Ji stance." Close your eyes and take deep breaths, focusing on your breath and relaxing your body.
2. Inhale deeply through your nose, raising your arms slowly to shoulder height with palms facing upward. Hold the position for a moment.
3. Exhale slowly through your mouth, lowering your arms back down to your sides. Focus on the sensation of relaxation as you breathe out.
4. Stand straight with your feet shoulder-width apart. Inhale and stretch your right arm overhead while bending your torso to the left. Hold for a few seconds. Return to the center and repeat on the other side.
5. Inhale as you raise both arms out to the sides and up overhead. Exhale as you bring your arms down in a circular motion, keeping the movement fluid and gentle.

6. End with a few moments in the Wu Ji stance, focusing on your breath and the energy within you. Feel the calm and balance you have cultivated.

Capoeira (Brazil)

Moving across continents to Brazil, we find Capoeira, an art form that seamlessly merges dance and martial arts. Originating from enslaved Africans, Capoeira was a survival mechanism disguised as dance, enabling practitioners to train in combat under the guise of rhythmical movements (Capoeira History, n.d.).

Today, it is celebrated as a form of martial art and a vibrant cultural expression that promotes community bonding and physical coordination. Practicing Capoeira requires agility, rhythm, and awareness, engaging your mind and body in dynamic harmony. Music, chants, and interactions among participants create a communal experience, allowing emotional release and enhancing social connections. Capoeira illustrates the power of movement as a unifying force, bridging physical discipline with cultural identity.

Below are simple Capoeira movements to try:

1. **Ginga**: The fundamental movement in Capoeira, a side-to-side rocking motion that helps build rhythm and balance. Practice shifting your weight from one foot to another and maintaining a low stance.
2. **Meia Lua de Frente**: A front crescent kick that can be executed from the ginga. Shift your weight onto one leg and swing the other leg in a circular motion, striking with the heel.
3. **Queixada**: Similar to the Meia Lua de Frente but with a diagonal kick that originates from the side. This kick is delivered with the heel and can be used to evade or strike an opponent.
4. **Negativa**: A low defense movement that involves lowering your body and placing one hand on the ground while bending the opposite knee. This allows you to evade attacks while staying low to the ground.

5. **Cocorinha**: A squat-like position that involves lowering your body while keeping your feet flat on the ground. This position helps to maintain a low center of gravity and is often used for evasion.
6. **Jogo**: Although not a single movement, practicing the flow and rhythm of Capoeira with a partner can help you apply basic movements in a playful context. Focus on fluidity and creativity in transitioning between movements.

Bharatanatyam (India)

Turning to India, Bharatanatyam is one of the ancient classical dance forms rich in symbolism and spirituality. It integrates elements such as expression (abhinaya), gesture (mudra), and controlled breathing to tell stories and evoke emotions (The Art of Symbolism: Bharatanatyam Mudras Decoded, 2024).

More than an art form, Bharatanatyam is a somatic practice that unites breath and movement, guiding practitioners toward mindfulness and emotional introspection. Performers often describe losing themselves in the performance, experiencing catharsis and spiritual enlightenment (Mahamenan, 2024). Through its disciplined yet expressive nature, Bharatanatyam encourages practitioners to explore their emotional depths, offering therapeutic benefits similar to modern-day mindfulness practices.

If you'd be interested in exploring this form of dance therapy, here are simple movements to practice:

1. **Namaskar (Salutation):** Stand with your feet together, hands in prayer position at your chest. Bow slightly while maintaining the hand position.
2. **Adavu - Tatta Melu:** Shift your weight to one foot while lifting the other foot and tapping it on the ground. Alternate feet and keep your arms in a graceful position.
3. **Adavu - Nattadavu:** Stand with your feet together. Step forward with one foot, keeping the heel high and knee bent. Bring the other foot forward and repeat.
4. **Hand gestures (Mudras):** Practice simple mudras like "Anjali" (prayer) and "Chakra" (circle). Create a circle with

your fingers and thumbs, symbolizing the cyclical nature of life and energy.

5. **Bharatanatyam stance (Araimandi):** Bend your knees deeply and keep your feet flat on the ground. This position helps with balance and core strength.
6. **Basic turns (Vrittis):** Practice slow turns on your feet, focusing on posture and maintaining a strong core.
7. **Simple expressions (Abhinaya):** Look in a mirror and practice expressing basic emotions through your facial expressions and hand movements.

Aikido (Japan)

Aikido is a Japanese martial art known for its focus on harmony and fluidity of movement. Unlike many other martial arts, Aikido teaches its practitioners to defend themselves while matching the opponent's energy (Aikido: The Martial Art of Harmony and Non-Resistance, 2023). This art emphasizes balance, both physical and emotional, and encourages practitioners to learn to stay centered and calm, even in challenging situations.

As students practice Aikido, they improve their physical skills and also work on healthy conflict resolution and emotional regulation, learning to remain composed and focused under pressure. This harmony can translate into everyday life. Aikido helps individuals respond to stress more effectively by promoting inner balance and peace (Aikido: The Martial Art of Harmony and Non-Resistance, 2023).

Here are beginner-friendly Aikido movements you can practice:

1. **Tai Sabaki (Body movement):** Practice moving your body in all directions. Focus on stepping forward, backward, and sideways while maintaining your balance.
2. **Tenkan (turning):** Stand with your feet shoulder-width apart. Rotate your body 180 degrees to face the opposite direction, keeping your feet in place.
3. **Kuzushi (Balance breaking):** Partner with a family member or practice with an imaginary partner. Gently push against their shoulder while maintaining your own stability.

4. **Shomen Uchi (Overhead strike):** Practice this movement by raising your arms above your head and striking downward, simulating an attack. Focus on fluid movement and proper stance.

5. **Katate Dori (One-hand grab):** Imagine someone grabbing your wrist. Practice stepping back and turning your body in response to the grab to release yourself.

6. **Irimi (Entering movement):** Simulate entering into an opponent's space by stepping forward decisively without compromising your balance.

7. **Atemi (Striking):** Practice basic punching motions, emphasizing precision and control.

8. **Zanshin (Awareness):** Spend time in a standing position, practicing awareness of your surroundings. Shift your weight and breathe deeply.

Glastonbury Medicine Wheel

The Glastonbury Medicine Wheel is a practice rooted in Celtic traditions. It uses the natural elements of earth, air, fire, and water as symbols to connect the body and spirit. Each element represents a different aspect of life and can guide you in your personal journey (The Celtic Medicine Wheel's Spiritual Links to Indigenous Traditions, 2024).

During a session that utilizes the Medicine Wheel, you might start by focusing on the element of earth and practice grounding exercises, like feeling your feet on the ground, to promote stability. Next, you may move on to the element of air, practicing breathwork to clear your mind. The fire element can be explored through movement that embodies passion and energy, while water might emphasize fluidity and emotional release. By experiencing each element, you can gain insights into your life and promote a sense of wholeness. The guided movement throughout this process builds a deeper connection between the body and spirit, leading to personal growth and healing.

Here is an example of a typical Medicine Wheel session where all four elements are explored for mind-body integration:

Begin your session by finding a comfortable space where you can connect with nature and the elements. As you stand in this space, take a moment to observe your surroundings, allowing yourself to become fully present.

1. **Earth:** Start by focusing on the Earth element. Imagine yourself standing firmly on the ground. Visualize roots extending from your feet deep into the Earth, anchoring you. Take a moment to appreciate the support and stability that the Earth provides. Reflect on what grounding means to you and how it aids in your overall well-being.

2. **Water:** Next, turn your attention to the Water element. Find a small bowl or container filled with water. Sit comfortably and gently touch the surface of the water, noticing its coolness and fluidity. As you dip your fingers in, imagine each drop representing your emotions. Allow yourself to express any feelings or thoughts that rise to the surface. Consider how water flows freely and how this can inspire you to navigate your own emotional landscape.

3. **Fire:** Now, introduce the Fire element. Light a small candle or sit near a safe fire source. Observe the flames as they dance and flicker. Think about the transformative power of fire in your life. What passions and desires are ignited within you? Take a few moments to visualize your aspirations burning bright, fueling your motivation and energy.

4. **Air:** Finally, embrace the Air element. Find a spot where you can feel the breeze or, if indoors, imagine the sensation of fresh air entering your space. With each inhale, envision breathing in clarity and inspiration. With each exhale, let go of any tension or negativity. Reflect on how the Air element connects you to communication and expression and consider what messages you want to share with the world.

As you integrate these four elements, conclude your activity by sitting in silence for a few moments, feeling the balance and harmony within your mind and body. Embrace the connection you have established with each element.

Huna

Huna is a philosophy from Hawaii that explores the connection between physical and spiritual well-being. This system includes various practices that involve breath and body movement (James, 2017). It teaches individuals how to align their physical health with their spiritual needs, promoting overall wellness.

Practicing Huna might involve simple techniques, such as focusing on deep breathing; as you breathe in, you might visualize drawing in positive energy, and as you exhale, you can imagine releasing negativity.

Additionally, Huna can incorporate movements that promote energy flow within the body, such as gentle exercises to enhance physical health while simultaneously tuning into our spiritual selves.

Here are some Huna practices that are simple yet effective for aligning your physical and spiritual well-being:

1. **Breath work (Ha breath):** Engage in deep, intentional breathing to connect with your inner self. Inhale deeply, filling your lungs, and exhale slowly, visualizing releasing any tension or negativity.
2. **Aloha spirit:** Embrace the concept of Aloha, which includes love, compassion, and kindness. Cultivate a mindset of gratitude and connection with yourself and others, creating harmony in both body and spirit.
3. **Ho'oponopono:** Practice this Hawaiian forgiveness ritual to release emotional burdens. Recite the phrases *"I'm sorry, please forgive me, thank you, I love you"* to heal relationships and align your spirit with positivity.
4. **Mana and energy work:** Focus on channeling your life force energy (mana) through physical exercises like hula or tai chi. Visualize this energy flowing freely, promoting physical vitality and spiritual balance.
5. **Nature connection:** Spend time in nature, whether through hiking, swimming, or simply meditating outdoors. Connect with the earth's energy to revitalize your physical and spiritual state.

Across cultures, somatic practices remind us that healing is a shared human experience that transcends boundaries. Though the movements, rituals, and philosophies may differ, they all point to the same truth: the body holds wisdom, and through it, we can find balance and connection. Exploring these traditions helps you see that healing isn't confined to one method or culture; it's a living dialogue between body, mind, and spirit, inviting you to come home to yourself in new and meaningful ways.

Case Studies of Somatic Therapy in Diverse Populations

Somatic therapy takes many forms depending on who's practicing it and the community it serves. Culture, language, and tradition shape how people relate to the body and approach healing. When these influences are acknowledged and included, therapy becomes more meaningful and accessible. The following stories show how somatic healing can be adapted in ways that respect cultural values and deepen connection.

Latino Communities

In many Latino families, healing is a shared experience. Family connection isn't just encouraged, it's essential. When Maria, a young mother, began somatic therapy to manage her anxiety, she was hesitant at first. But everything changed when her therapist invited her family to take part in a few sessions.

Sharing stories about health and wellness within her cultural context helped her feel seen and supported. As her loved ones joined her in learning body-awareness practices, Maria's sense of belonging grew stronger. The process became less about treatment and more about collective healing rooted in family and trust.

African American Perspectives

For many African American clients, the path to healing is often intertwined with generational and systemic trauma. James, a middle-aged man living with symptoms of PTSD, began exploring body-centered therapy that recognized both his personal and ancestral experiences.

His sessions included rhythmic movement and grounding through breath, often paired with music that resonated with his cultural roots. These familiar sounds and motions helped him release tension that words alone couldn't reach. Healing, in this sense, became not only personal but also a way to reclaim strength from a lineage that had endured so much.

Asian Cultural Contexts

In Asian traditions, the link between body, energy, and emotion has long been understood through philosophies such as Qi and Yin-Yang balance. When Mei, a young woman from a Chinese background, sought somatic therapy for stress, her experience deepened when her therapist integrated familiar movement practices inspired by Tai Chi and Qigong.

The language of energy flow helped her make sense of her body's signals in a way that felt natural. By blending ancient wisdom with modern techniques, her sessions became a bridge between tradition and self-awareness.

Shared Threads of Healing

Across all cultures, one theme shines through: people heal best when their values, families, and traditions are honored in the process. Whether it's including family members, recognizing ancestral pain, or incorporating familiar spiritual practices, somatic therapy thrives when it respects the unique story each person brings. Healing, after all, is not just about the body; it's about belonging

Key Takeaways

- Cultural backgrounds profoundly shape the understanding and use of somatic therapy, incorporating diverse beliefs and practices into healing journeys. Through indigenous rituals, Eastern mindfulness, communal African approaches, and more, each culture offers a unique lens on body-mind connections.
- These traditions remind us that healing is not only about addressing physical symptoms but also nurturing spiritual and community bonds. By embracing these ideas, you can find deeper meaning and support in your therapeutic experiences, enhancing your emotional resilience and strengthening a sense of belonging.
- As global interest in holistic therapies grows, there's power in combining ancient wisdom with contemporary techniques, creating personalized healing paths. Therapists can integrate cultural perspectives into their practices to ensure accessibility and cultivate empowerment for those seeking healing.

Healing is most powerful when it's viewed through an expansive lens, one that honors who we are, where we come from, and the stories that have shaped us. When culture, ancestry, and personal experience are embraced rather than overlooked, somatic work becomes more than a method; it becomes a return to wholeness.

In the next chapter, we'll explore practical somatic exercises designed to help you build and nurture positive, supportive relationships, because healing within ourselves naturally extends to how we connect with others.

06.

Navigating Relationships Through Somatic Awareness

Your task is not to seek for love, but merely to seek and find all the barriers within yourself that you have built against it. –Rumi

“

Relationships can be some of our greatest teachers. They show us where we feel safe, where we shut down, and where old wounds still live beneath the surface. When we start paying attention to what our bodies are telling us in those moments, tightness in the chest, a lump in the throat, a sudden rush of heat, we begin to see how deeply our emotional and physical worlds are connected.

Somatic awareness helps us notice these signals before they spiral into conflict or disconnection. It gives us a way to understand our patterns; the ways we pull closer, push away, or lose ourselves trying to keep the peace. In this chapter, we'll explore how tuning into your body can reshape the way you relate to others, build emotional safety, and create boundaries that feel healthy rather than heavy.

Recognizing Emotional Patterns in Relationships

You've probably noticed that certain interactions seem to push the same emotional buttons again and again. Maybe it's a tone of voice, a familiar argument, or the feeling of not being heard. These moments aren't random; they're cues from your body pointing toward something deeper.

Somatic awareness helps you catch these signals before they take over. When you start noticing where tension rises or where your energy drops in specific relationships, you begin to understand the emotional patterns running beneath the surface. In the pages ahead, we'll explore gentle exercises to help you identify these patterns, understand what your body is communicating, and begin shifting how you show up in your connections.

Tracing Emotional Triggers and Their Origin

Emotional patterns are not just arbitrary; they often stem from your past experiences. Your history, particularly traumatic events, can significantly influence how you behave today. For instance, if you have experienced abandonment, you may find it challenging to trust your partner fully. This underlying fear can manifest in jealousy or constant reassurance-seeking. Realizing that your past traumas impact your present behaviors enables you to dissect conflicts more clearly.

One way to understand how your past traumas impact your current relationships is to identify possible emotional triggers and trace where they come from. Emotional triggers are irrational responses to situations that remind you of painful memories. While these reactions seem uncalled for, they provide clues about unresolved emotional issues you may be holding onto.

The following exercise will help you identify emotional triggers and reflect on where they might stem from.

Instructions

1. Select one specific close relationship you would like to focus on for this exercise. Think about situations in this relationship that evoke strong emotional reactions in you (positive or negative). Reflect on at least three specific instances where you felt a strong emotional response. Reflect on what happened and how you felt.

____

____

2. What specific words, actions, or behaviors from the other person trigger an emotional response in you?

3. How do you typically react when you experience these triggers? Is it a fight, flight, or freeze response?

4. Can you identify any patterns or recurring themes in these emotional triggers? Have you experienced similar feelings in other relationships or past experiences?

5. Can you trace these emotional triggers back to childhood experiences or past traumas?

6. What beliefs or assumptions do you hold about yourself or your relationship that might contribute to these triggers?

____

____

____

____

____

____

7. Document your insights by creating a chart or mind map that visually represents your emotional triggers and their possible origins. Use different colors to signify different types of emotions (e.g., anger, sadness, joy) and draw connections to where these emotions might stem from.
8. If comfortable, share your findings with a trusted friend or a therapist. Discuss how recognizing these triggers can impact your relationship moving forward.

Creating a New Narrative

Reframing emotional narratives provides a powerful tool for transformation. By changing the story you tell yourself about your emotions, you can shift your perspectives and, consequently, your interactions. If you view yourself as inherently unlovable due to past rejections, every minor conflict may feel like proof of this narrative. However, by questioning these narratives and exploring alternative perspectives, you empower yourself to alter your response to relational challenges. This process begins with asking: *"Is my perception based on current reality or rooted in past insecurities?"*

Challenging existing beliefs about yourself isn't easy, particularly when you are still harboring anger, guilt, or shame about past experiences. However, with a compassionate approach, you can begin to unlearn negative perspectives and feed your mind empowering stories about yourself and others.

Here is a nonjudgmental inner-child exercise to help you create new narratives about yourself in relation to others:

1. Imagine a younger version of yourself, perhaps as you were at around six or seven years old. Observe your emotions, your expressions, and how you carry yourself.
2. In your mind, gently ask your inner child how they feel about relationships with others. Listen to their responses without judgment. Acknowledge their fears, insecurities, and beliefs.
3. Think about the harmful narratives you've adopted over time. For each negative belief, create a positive counternarrative. For example, if you think, *"I am not worthy of love,"* reframe it to *"I am deserving of love and respect."*
4. Take a moment to address your inner child, offering understanding and compassion. Share the positive narratives you want them to embrace. Encourage them to let go of the old beliefs and accept the new empowering ones.

As you practice creating new narratives, remember that change doesn't happen all at once. The stories you've carried were built over years of experience and protection, and rewriting them takes time and tenderness.

Each moment you pause to question an old belief, every time you choose compassion instead of criticism, you're building a new foundation for connection, both with yourself and with others. Healing doesn't erase the past; it reshapes your relationship to it, allowing you to meet life and love from a place of greater peace and self-trust.

The next step is learning to bring this awareness into your daily interactions. Mindfulness helps you stay present when old stories resurface, giving you the space to respond instead of react.

Practicing Mindfulness in Relationship Dynamics

Mindfulness helps us stay present in the moments that test us most. It gives us a way to notice what's happening inside before reacting to what's happening outside. Think about a time when you felt hurt or dismissed in a conversation. The natural impulse might be to argue, withdraw, or shut down, but mindfulness invites a small pause.

In that pause, you can take a breath and feel what's really there. Maybe it's an old fear surfacing, or a need to feel understood. When you give yourself a moment to notice instead of react, something shifts. You begin to respond with more clarity and compassion, both for yourself and for the other person. With practice, this awareness brings more ease into your relationships and opens space for healthier, more honest connection.

When emotions run high, it can be easy to lose your footing in the moment. Having a simple way to ground yourself can make all the difference. One approach I often use is the *CALM* method, a mindful framework you can use anytime tension starts to rise.

CALM stands for ***C**heck-In*, ***A**cknowledge*, ***L**isten*, and ***M**indfully Respond*. These four steps help you stay present during conflict so you can engage thoughtfully rather than react impulsively. Let's walk through them together.

Step 1: Check-In

Begin by checking in with yourself. Take a moment to assess your emotional state and physical sensations. Try to recognize what you are feeling so that you can make sense of your emotional experience.

For example, you might acknowledge: *"I'm feeling really frustrated right now. I need to take a moment to breathe before we continue this conversation."*

____

____

____

____

____

____

Step 2: Acknowledge

Acknowledge your feelings and the other person's emotions. Validating emotions can diffuse tension. Remember that validation isn't the same as agreement. It involves accepting another person's perspective and showing them that you care.

For example, when you are validating someone, you can say: *"I understand that you're feeling hurt by what I said, and I can see how that would upset you."*

____

____

Step 3: Listen

Practice active listening. Really focus on what the other person is saying without planning your response while they talk. Active listening involves using nonverbal cues like maintaining eye contact, nodding, and turning your body toward the speaker. However, it can also include language that conveys that you are listening.

Practice different ways of communicating that you are listening. For example, you could say: *"I'm here to listen to your perspective. Please tell me more about how you feel and what led to this disagreement."*

Step 4: Mindfully Respond

After processing the conversation, respond mindfully. Consider your words carefully and aim for a constructive outcome. Pay attention to your tone and choice of words, making sure that they don't come across defensive or combative. Essentially, respond in a manner that would make you feel understood.

For example, a mindful response could be: *"I appreciate you sharing your feelings with me. How can we work together to find a solution that feels good for both of us?"*

Using Body Awareness to Enhance Communication

In today's fast-paced world, we often rush through conversations without realizing how much we're communicating beyond words. Our posture, tone, and facial expressions speak volumes, even when we're silent. When you start paying attention to these subtle signals in yourself and others, something shifts. You begin to hear what isn't being said, to sense emotion beneath the surface, and to respond with greater empathy and understanding.

Body awareness helps you slow down enough to notice these cues and use them to strengthen your connections. Before we move into a few body awareness exercises, let's look at a simple example of how nonverbal signals can shape a conversation.

Consider two friends sharing a conversation. One is speaking animatedly about a recent personal struggle while the other listens, nodding occasionally but appearing distracted. Their posture tells its own story: arms crossed, leaning slightly away. These nonverbal cues may unintentionally convey disinterest or judgment, potentially leading to misunderstanding or hurt feelings. By becoming aware of these signals, both people can adjust their body language and create a more supportive, empathetic exchange.

Assertive Body Language

Being assertive isn't about being forceful; it's about being clear, grounded, and respectful in how you express yourself. It means saying what you feel and need without dismissing anyone else's experience. When your words and body language match, when your tone, posture, and gestures align with your message, you communicate with confidence.

Notice how your body feels when you're being direct yet kind. Your shoulders relax, your breath steadies, and your voice feels more even. This is assertiveness in action: open, steady, and self-assured. The more you practice it, the easier it becomes to express yourself honestly without fear of conflict or judgment, creating space for clearer communication and genuine understanding.

The table below highlights the differences between assertive, passive, and aggressive body language. Take a few moments to look it over, then reflect on your recent interactions with friends, family, or colleagues.

Body Language Type	**Characteristics**
Assertive	maintains good eye contact
	open posture (arms and legs uncrossed)
	calm, steady tone of voice
	uses gestures for emphasis
	faces the person directly
	confident facial expressions
	takes up space without being dominant
Passive	avoids eye contact
	closed posture (arms and legs crossed)
	quiet, soft voice
	minimal gestures
	faced away from the person
	uncertain facial expressions
	stands or sits in a small space
Aggressive	piercing or glaring eye contact
	closed and tense posture
	loud, harsh tone of voice
	wild or dominating gestures
	leans in too close or gets into personal space
	intimidating facial expressions
	takes up space aggressively

Reflection Questions

1. In what ways do I position my body and movement when interacting with friends, and how might this influence the dynamics of our conversations?

2. How freely do I express my emotions through body language around family members, and what underlying factors shape this comfort or discomfort?

3. What specific differences can I identify in my posture when I'm with colleagues as opposed to being with family or friends, and what might these differences say about my feelings in each context?

4. Do I notice a shift in the softness of my tone when I communicate with certain individuals, and how does this reflect my emotional comfort and connection with them?

5. During potentially confrontational encounters, do I tend to exhibit assertive or aggressive body language, and what messages am I trying to convey through these body movements?

6. In what ways do my habitual body language tendencies influence the quality and nature of my relationships with others, both positively and negatively?

7. What specific nonverbal cues do I observe in the body language of others that shape my impressions and judgments of them, and how does this affect my interactions?

As you explore these reflections, remember that communication is a living exchange; your body and energy are always part of the conversation. Each time you notice yourself shifting from passive or aggressive tendencies toward a more open, balanced stance, you strengthen your confidence and deepen your connection with others.

Setting Intentions for Positive Interactions

Before every meaningful conversation, there's a small moment of choice, how you want to show up, what energy you want to bring, and what outcome you hope to create. Taking a moment to set an intention helps you anchor this choice in awareness.

Imagine walking into a conversation that might be challenging. Instead of bracing yourself for conflict, you pause, breathe, and decide how you want to engage, perhaps with openness, curiosity, or compassion. This simple act shifts everything. Your body softens, your tone steadies, and you naturally become more receptive. Approaching interactions this way invites understanding instead of tension and helps create the kind of connection both people can feel.

The following intention-setting exercise will prepare you for positive engagements with others. Regardless of the nature of the conversation, you will step in feeling confident about the interaction.

Instructions

1. Spend a moment to deeply contemplating the upcoming conversation. Create a vivid mental image of a positive outcome where you communicate with clarity and confidence, while the other person responds with openness and positivity. Allow yourself to feel the energy of this successful interaction.
2. Choose a powerful affirmation that resonates with your goals for the interaction, such as *"I embrace understanding and connection with others,"* or *"I listen with compassion and articulate my thoughts with clarity."* Repeat this affirmation silently, letting it sink into your consciousness.
3. Reflect on the emotions you wish to cultivate during and after the conversation. Identify feelings such as respect, empathy, and joy. Use this list as a beacon, reminding yourself to embody these empowering emotions throughout the interaction.
4. Think of three aspects of yourself and your abilities that you genuinely appreciate. Recognizing these qualities will significantly boost your self-confidence and establish a positive atmosphere as you engage in conversation.
5. As you prepare for the engagement, focus on embodying openness, approachability, and curiosity. Create a mindset that welcomes learning and growth from the conversation, embracing the potential for deeper understanding.
6. Just before entering the interaction, take a deep breath to center yourself. Take a moment to mentally affirm your intention one last time, allowing it to guide your thoughts and actions as you step forward into the conversation.

Applying these body awareness principles in everyday scenarios can be transformative. For instance, in workplace settings, where communication is key to collaboration, you, who are mindful of nonverbal cues and body language, can help create an inclusive and cooperative environment. You, as a leader who practices active listening and sets clear intentions when addressing your teams, are more likely to inspire trust and loyalty, resulting in higher morale and productivity.

Similarly, in your personal relationships, these skills can bridge gaps in understanding and resolve conflicts more effectively. You and your partner, who prioritize body awareness in your interactions, are better equipped to navigate disagreements compassionately, focusing on solutions rather than assigning blame. Recognizing emotional states can prevent unnecessary escalations, allowing you to reconnect and reaffirm your commitment to each other.

Ultimately, somatic awareness in communication invites you to look inward as much as outward. By becoming more conscious of your own nonverbal cues and emotional patterns, you begin to understand what drives your reactions and responses. This awareness allows you to communicate with greater honesty and calm, strengthening trust and connection in all your relationships.

As you deepen this awareness, the next step is learning how to use it to honor your personal limits and emotional space.

Practicing Boundary-Setting With Somatic Tools

Healthy boundaries are the foundation of balanced relationships. They protect your energy, honor your needs, and help you stay connected to yourself while still caring for others. Think of them as the space where your wellbeing can breathe, a gentle but firm line that keeps you from becoming emotionally drained or overextended.

When boundaries are unclear, it's easy to feel pulled in every direction, giving more than you have to give. Noticing where this happens is the first step toward change. Somatic awareness can help by tuning you into the signals your body sends when a boundary is being crossed: tension in your shoulders, a tightness in your chest, or a heaviness in your gut. The following techniques will help you strengthen this awareness and create boundaries that feel both compassionate and firm.

Somatic Boundary Identification

Often, your body holds the answers to unrecognized limits, manifesting discomfort or tension when boundaries are crossed. For instance, you might feel a knot in your stomach when agreeing to something you genuinely don't have time for, signaling an internal conflict with your boundaries. Through somatic listening, you can attune to these physical signals, using them as guides to identify and articulate your limits more effectively.

One practical method for boundary identification involves paying attention to any areas of tension or discomfort, noting what circumstances trigger these feelings. As patterns emerge, they provide insight into your personal boundaries and the situations in which they need to be reinforced. Here is an activity that you can practice.

Instructions

1. Close your eyes and take a few deep breaths. Inhale through your nose, allowing your belly to expand, and exhale slowly through your mouth. Repeat this for 3–5 breaths.
2. Starting from the top of your head, slowly bring your awareness down through your body. Notice any areas of tension, discomfort, or tightness. Spend a few moments on each part of your body—head, shoulders, chest, abdomen, arms, legs, and feet.
3. As you notice areas of tension or discomfort, ask yourself questions like:
   - What does this sensation feel like (sharp, dull, tight)?
   - Where is it located in my body?
   - Is it constant, or does it come and go?
4. Think about situations or experiences that might have led to these physical cues. Consider past interactions, environments, or specific events.

5. For each physical cue you identified, label it. Ask yourself:
    - What boundary might this sensation be related to?
    - Is it a physical boundary (personal space), emotional boundary (how others treat you), or relational boundary (level of intimacy)?

6. After you have identified and labeled your sensations, take a few moments to reflect on what you have learned about your boundaries. Consider journaling your insights or discussing them with a trusted friend or therapist

Make this somatic listening activity a regular practice to deepen your understanding of your personal boundaries and enhance your self-awareness. It's important to approach this activity with self-compassion and patience, recognizing that boundary-setting is a personal journey that evolves over time.

Communicating Your Boundaries With Compassion

Once your boundaries are identified, communicating them effectively is essential. This requires clear, compassionate dialogue that honors both your needs and the other person's perspective. Somatic practices can support this communication process by encouraging calmness and confidence. Before initiating a conversation about boundaries, practicing deep breathing or engaging in a brief meditation can help center your emotions, allowing you to communicate more clearly and empathetically.

Here is a compassion meditation to help you recognize the significance of your boundaries while respecting the humanity of those whom you are setting boundaries with.

Script

1. Close your eyes gently and take a deep breath in through your nose, filling your lungs completely. Hold for a moment and then exhale slowly through your mouth. Let any tension, stress, or worries drift away with your breath.

2. As you settle into a relaxed state, bring your attention to your body. Notice how it feels in this moment. Acknowledge any sensations, emotions, or thoughts that arise, accepting them without judgment.

3. Visualize a soft, warm light surrounding you. This light represents your compassion and love. With every inhalation, imagine this light expanding, enveloping you in a gentle embrace and reminding you of your worth and the importance of honoring your own needs.

4. Reflect on a situation where you feel the need to set a boundary. Picture it clearly in your mind. Acknowledge the

feelings that arise—whether it's discomfort, fear, or uncertainty—and honor those feelings as valid.

5. In this space of compassion, remind yourself that it is perfectly acceptable to protect your energy and well-being. Think about how healthy boundaries are not just about saying "no" but about saying "yes" to yourself and your needs.
6. Focus on the other person involved in this situation. Visualize them standing before you, surrounded by a warm light as well. Recognize their humanity, their struggles, and their needs.
7. With an open heart, silently express your desire to communicate your boundaries with respect and kindness. Imagine the conversation flowing naturally, where both your needs and theirs are acknowledged and honored.
8. As you continue to breathe deeply, repeat these affirmations in your mind:
   - *"I am worthy of respect and care."*
   - *"My needs are important."*
   - *"I can express my boundaries with love and compassion."*
9. Take a moment to visualize the outcome of this conversation. Feel the relief and empowerment that comes from honoring your needs while respecting the other person.
10. When you feel ready, slowly bring your attention back to your breath and gently open your eyes. Carry this feeling of compassion with you as you move through your day, ready to express your boundaries with clarity and kindness.

Think of your boundaries like a garden. Each relationship, like every plant, needs different care at different stages of growth. Somatic awareness helps you stay attuned to these natural shifts, noticing when something needs more space or a little extra tending. If a boundary starts to feel tight or uncomfortable, it may be a sign that it's time to adjust it. Revisiting and refining your boundaries as you grow allows your relationships to evolve with greater understanding and connection.

As you continue developing this awareness, you can begin to apply it in more intimate spaces of connection and trust.

Somatic Exercises to Enhance Romantic Relationships

In romantic relationships, it is important to connect not just mentally but also physically and emotionally. One way to strengthen this bond is through somatic exercises. These activities help you and your partner become more aware of your bodies and how they interact with each other. By practicing these exercises, you can enhance empathy, communication, and emotional connections.

Partnered Mirroring

One effective somatic exercise is partnered mirror work. This exercise involves standing in front of each other and reflecting each other's nonverbal cues and body language. For instance, if one partner raises their hand, the other should do the same at the same time. This exercise encourages you to observe and respond to each other with greater understanding.

To practice mirroring with a partner, follow these steps:

1. Dedicate 10–15 minutes for the exercise, allowing you to disconnect from distractions such as mobile devices or external noises. This period can be enhanced by finding a quiet, serene environment that increases concentration.
2. Begin by sitting or standing a comfortable distance apart—about an arm's length. Ensure both of you have enough personal space to feel at ease. Engage in a brief conversation about the purpose of the exercise and share any initial feelings or intentions to create a supportive atmosphere.
3. As you start, establish consistent eye contact. This connection is important for empathy and attunement. Try to understand each other's physical movements and emotional expressions. For example, if your partner smiles, replicate the smile to create a sense of unity.
4. Pay close attention to the subtle movements of your partner. If they lean forward, you should do the same in a synchronized manner. This can be deepened further by observing their gestures—if one partner raises their hand, the other

should lift their hand similarly, creating a fluid exchange of body language.

5. After some initial movements, introduce gentle verbal cues such as *"I notice you're feeling energetic"* or *"I sense you're a bit reserved."* Respond by mimicking the message and tone—a soft tone for calm emotions, or an excited tone for happy expressions.
6. Encourage each other to change the pace or intensity of your movements. For instance, one partner can start at a slow pace and increase speed gradually. The other partner should follow suit, allowing for creative exploration within the mirroring.
7. After about 5–7 minutes, switch roles and allow the other partner to lead the mirroring exercise.
8. At the end of the exercise, take a few minutes to share reflections. Discuss how it felt to mirror each other, what insights were gained, and how body language can affect communication.

Partnered mirroring offers more than a shared physical experience; it builds trust, empathy, and emotional resonance. As you learn to move together, you begin to sense each other's rhythms and unspoken feelings. This practice also helps you stay present, deepening not only your awareness of your partner but also your understanding of yourself within the relationship.

Embodied Communication

Another valuable practice is embodied communication. This involves using body movements to express thoughts or feelings instead of relying solely on words. Choose one interaction each day to communicate without speaking. For example, if you are happy, you might jump or dance a little. If you are feeling sad, you could slump your shoulders or move slowly.

During this exercise, pay attention to how your partner responds to your movements. This will help both of you notice the nonverbal signals that often go unnoticed. You can also take turns leading and following, which helps cultivate trust and understanding. After your session, share how you felt during the exercise and any insights gained.

Practicing embodied communication reminds you that so much of connection happens beyond words. By expressing emotion through movement, you open a channel for deeper understanding and playfulness in your relationship. This kind of shared awareness strengthens emotional intimacy and helps you stay attuned to one another's unspoken experiences.

Movement and Emotion Reflection

Exploring movement practices like dance or yoga can be very beneficial for connecting physical sensations with emotional states. The idea here is to pay attention to how specific movements make you feel. For instance, during a dance session, notice if certain rhythms bring up joy or sadness.

To integrate this practice, set up a time once a week to engage in a movement activity together. Choose an environment that is comfortable and safe. It could be a dance class, a yoga session, or even just playing music at home. As you move, reflect on how different emotions arise within your body. This can lead to valuable insights about how emotions manifest physically. After the session, discuss what you experienced, how certain movements related to your feelings, and whether any emotions were difficult to express.

Regularly exploring movement and emotion together helps you recognize how energy and feeling flow through your body and relationships. The more you pay attention to these subtle shifts, the easier it becomes to sense when emotions need expression, grounding, or release. This shared awareness nurtures balance, connection, and a deeper sense of emotional understanding between you and your partner.

As you continue developing this awareness through movement, another meaningful way to strengthen connection is through touch, the most direct and immediate form of embodied communication.

Intentional Touch

Intentional touch is a mindful way to connect with your partner through physical presence and care. It's less about technique and more about slowing down, paying attention, and feeling fully present in the moment. This can be as simple as holding hands, hugging, or offering a gentle massage. What matters most is the *quality* of your attention, the warmth, curiosity, and openness you bring to the experience.

To practice:

1. **Begin with consent and conversation.** Take a few minutes to talk about what kind of touch feels comfortable and supportive for both of you. This sets the tone for safety and trust.
2. **Create a calm environment.** Choose a quiet space and set aside time when you won't be interrupted. You might dim the lights, play soft music, or simply sit together in silence before beginning.
3. **Start with grounding.** Take a few slow breaths together to settle your energy. Notice the rhythm of your breathing and the feeling of your feet or body supported by the floor or surface beneath you.
4. **Engage in gentle touch.** Begin with a simple gesture, perhaps holding hands or placing a hand on your partner's shoulder. As you touch, focus on the sensations: warmth, texture, movement, and breath. Notice any changes in your body, heart rate, or emotions.
5. **Stay present and responsive.** Let the experience unfold naturally. If you sense tension, pause and take a breath together. If something feels especially soothing, stay with it a little longer. You might alternate who gives and who receives touch, keeping the exchange mutual and attentive.
6. **Reflect together.** When you're finished, take a few moments to share what you noticed, physically, emotionally, and energetically. Discuss what felt nurturing or surprising, and express gratitude for the shared experience.

Taking time to practice these exercises together strengthens the bond between you. Each moment of shared awareness, whether through movement, touch, or simple presence, builds trust and emotional safety. The goal here is connection. As you continue exploring somatic practices within your relationship, notice how these small, intentional acts create more ease, tenderness, and understanding between you.

Key Takeaways

- Becoming more attuned to your emotional patterns and physical responses allows you to gain valuable insights into how past traumas influence current behaviors. This awareness allows you to interact with others more thoughtfully, leading to deeper connections and encouraging personal growth.
- Additionally, somatic practices aid in identifying assertive body language and reinforcing personal boundaries. Mindfulness exercises, intention-setting, and body scanning help you become more present within yourself, providing crucial signals about where boundaries need to be set or adjusted.

As you strengthen your ability to communicate and connect through somatic awareness, it's equally important to bring that same level of presence back to yourself. Relationships thrive when we have the inner capacity to stay grounded, centered, and emotionally nourished. Caring for your own well-being is what allows you to show up fully for others without losing yourself in the process.

When I was recovering from breast cancer, I learned this truth in a very personal way. My body demanded attention, rest, and compassion in a way I had never experienced before. It wasn't only about physical healing; it was about rebuilding trust with my body and honoring what it needed moment by moment.

In the next chapter, I'll share some of the somatic self-care practices that supported me most during that time, gentle ways to restore energy, release tension, and reconnect with yourself on every level.

07.

Incorporating Self-Care and Somatic Practice

Within you there is a stillness and a sanctuary to which you can retreat at any time and be yourself. –Hermann Hesse

"

When life feels full and fast, self-care can easily fall to the bottom of the list. For me, it once felt like a luxury, something I'd get to "when things slowed down." But after recovering from breast cancer, I realized how essential it truly is. Self-care isn't pampering; it's how we maintain balance, peace of mind, and emotional steadiness.

Somatic practices make this process even more meaningful. By paying attention to your body's sensations: the tightness in your chest after a long day, the lightness that comes with movement, the calm that follows a deep breath, you start to understand what your body is asking for. These small moments of awareness open the door to healing and growth. In this chapter, we'll explore simple ways to integrate somatic awareness into everyday life so that caring for yourself becomes natural, nourishing, and deeply restorative.

Designing a Personalized Somatic Self-Care Plan

Creating a self-care plan that truly supports you starts with understanding your own needs. Your body, emotions, and life experiences are uniquely yours; what restores one person might not work for another. Honoring your individuality is key.

Take a moment to think about the different areas of your life, your emotional well-being, physical health, and daily responsibilities. Each plays a role in how balanced and energized you feel. In the next few pages, we'll explore practical ways to design a self-care plan that fits your lifestyle and helps you stay connected to what your body and mind need most.

Assessing Your Daily Needs

When you begin creating your self-care plan, start by looking closely at what makes your life unique. Notice the emotional patterns and physical demands that shape your days. Maybe you often feel anxious and need moments of calm to steady your breath, or perhaps you live with chronic pain and find relief through gentle stretching or restorative yoga. Paying attention to these personal rhythms helps you choose somatic practices that truly support you; ones that meet you where you are and nurture what you most need right now.

Here's a simple reflection to help you tune in to what you actually need each day. Think of it as your starting point for creating a self-care plan that truly fits your life.

1. Spend 5–10 minutes each evening reflecting on your day. Notice what activities made you feel energized and what left you feeling drained.

2. Break down your daily needs into categories: physical, emotional, social, spiritual, and mental. Under each category, list specific needs or activities that fulfill them. For example:

- **Physical:** Exercise, adequate sleep, nutrition
- **Emotional:** Time for hobbies, journaling, talking to a friend
- **Social:** Connecting with others, family time
- **Spiritual:** Meditation, nature walks, reading
- **Mental:** Learning, puzzles, creative outlets

3. Reflect on which needs feel most important right now and rate each need on a scale of 1–5, with 1 being least important and 5 being most important. This will help prioritize your self-care activities.

4. Evaluate how much time you currently spend on each category daily. Are you dedicating enough time to your self-care needs?
5. Based on your assessment, choose two to three needs from each category that you would like to incorporate into your daily routine. Make sure your goals are realistic and achievable.
6. Think through a simple action plan and the specific steps you can take to meet these needs. Consider a general timeframe and how you might notice your progress over time.

At the end of each week, review your feelings and progress. Adjust your self-care plan as needed to better meet your evolving needs.

Setting Realistic Goals

Setting goals you can actually stick with makes all the difference in staying motivated. It's easy to dream big and then feel let down when progress doesn't happen fast enough. But when you break your goals into smaller, doable steps, you start to see results, and this builds confidence and momentum. Think of it like training for a marathon: you don't start with 26 miles, you start with one.

Here's a creative reflection activity that taps into your senses to help you set realistic goals for your daily self-care routine.

Materials You May Want to Use

- a large piece of paper or a canvas
- colored markers
- glue and scissors
- timer
- stickers and other decorative items you may need
- magazines for cutting out images

Instructions

1. Take a moment to focus on your five senses: sight, sound, touch, taste, and smell. Reflect on how each sense can play a role in your self-care.
2. Set a timer for 10 minutes to brainstorm. With your materials in front of you, think about enjoyable activities related to each sense that can help you respond to your self-care needs.
3. Divide the canvas or paper into five sections—one for each sense. Use markers, cut-out images, and stickers to represent the self-care activities related to each sense. For example, your board can end up looking like this:
    a. **Sight:** A beautiful painting or a calming nature scene for visual peace.
    b. **Sound:** Create a playlist of favorite songs or sounds that make you feel good.

   c. **Touch:** Illustrate cozy blankets, soft fabrics, or massage items that bring comfort.

   d. **Taste:** Include images of healthy foods or treats that you enjoy, representing nourishing meals.

   e. **Smell:** Collect scents like essential oils, flowers, or candles that promote relaxation.

4. After creating your sensory board, take a moment to reflect on the activities and choose a few you can realistically bring into your daily life.
5. Spend a few minutes reflecting on your goals. Are they achievable? Adjust them if necessary. Keep your self-care canvas visible as a constant reminder of your self-care intentions.

Taking time to visualize your self-care through your senses helps make it tangible. Every image, word, or symbol you've added to your canvas represents a small but meaningful way to nurture yourself. Keep it somewhere visible as a reminder that caring for your body and mind isn't a luxury, it's a daily practice that supports balance and well-being.

Committing to Daily Somatic Practices

Through Habit Stacking

Life's pace can be unpredictable, so it's essential for you to design a self-care routine that's flexible. Integrating somatic practices doesn't mean creating rigid schedules, but rather finding ways to embed them naturally into the ebb and flow of your day.

Habit stacking is a simple yet powerful way to make somatic practices part of your everyday life. It means linking a new habit to something you already do regularly, so it becomes part of your natural rhythm instead of feeling like another task.

The following guidelines will help you create habit stacks to integrate somatic practices into your existing daily routine.

Instructions

1. Begin by noticing daily habits you already do consistently. These might include brushing your teeth, having your morning coffee, or commuting to work.

2. Choose somatic practices you want to incorporate, such as deep breathing, stretching, or mindful walking. For each existing habit, think about how you can seamlessly add your chosen somatic practice. For example, after brushing your teeth, you might take a minute for deep breathing or follow your morning coffee with a few stretches.

3. Reflect on how your new habit aligns with or enhances the existing one. Would doing a brief stretch after your morning coffee make you feel more awake?

4. How can you make the new practice enjoyable or rewarding?

5. What potential obstacles might you face, and how can you address them?

Try out your habit stacks for a week. Afterward, reflect on how they felt and whether adjustments are needed to make them more effective or enjoyable. Remember to be flexible in your approach. If a particular stack doesn't work, feel free to change the order or the specific practices until you find what resonates with you.

The beauty of personalized self-care is that it's flexible, it grows and changes with you. As your life shifts, so do your needs, energy, and priorities. What supports you today might look different from what helped you yesterday, or what you'll need tomorrow. Staying open to adjusting your practices keeps them meaningful, sustainable, and aligned with where you are right now.

Ultimately, creating a self-care routine that truly supports you takes a bit of experimentation. There's no one-size-fits-all approach; what feels grounding for one person might not resonate for another. Exploring different somatic practices helps you discover what genuinely nourishes you, both emotionally and physically, so your routine feels like a natural extension of your well-being rather than a checklist.

Reflective Journaling for Tracking Progress

Journaling is one of the most effective ways to build self-awareness and notice your growth as you integrate somatic practices into daily life. It's more than a record of what you've done; it's a space to pause, reflect, and connect with how your body and emotions are responding over time. This reflective process also helps you stay consistent and intentional in your practice. Below are three simple journaling approaches you can use to make reflection a natural part of your day.

Create a Dedicated Journaling Space

Having a dedicated spot for journaling can make it easier to stay consistent. Picture a cozy corner in your home with a comfortable chair, a soft blanket, maybe a plant or a candle, something that feels calm and inviting. This little nook becomes your cue to slow down, breathe, and reconnect with yourself. It signals to your mind and body that it's time for reflection and self-care. Setting aside a space just for this purpose helps you treat journaling as a meaningful part of your daily routine.

Choosing a designated journaling space at home doesn't have to be difficult. Simply ensure you follow the guidelines below:

1. Find a space away from distractions such as television or noisy environments. A corner of your bedroom, a cozy nook in your living room, or even a spot in your garden can be ideal.
2. Make sure your chosen area is comfortable. Include a supportive chair, a soft cushion, or even a bean bag. A comfortable space encourages longer journaling sessions.
3. If possible, choose a place near a window. Natural light can enhance your mood and creativity. You can also add plants to breathe life into the space.
4. Ensure your journaling area is tidy. Use a small bookshelf or drawer to store your journals, pens, and other supplies. An organized space promotes clarity of thought.
5. Add items that inspire you, such as artwork, photographs, or quotes. Personalizing your space can make it feel more inviting and motivating.
6. Consider lighting options like a small lamp or candles. A tranquil atmosphere can set the right mood for reflection and creativity.
7. Communicate your journaling time to family or roommates to minimize disruptions. Setting boundaries promotes a focused journaling experience.
8. If you prefer variety, consider a portable journaling kit that you can move around your home. This way, you can switch up your location while keeping your supplies handy.

Prompting Self-Reflection With Guided Questions

Once you've created a space that feels calm and supportive, try using guided questions to help you reflect more deeply. These prompts are designed to help you notice what's happening within you, to explore your emotions, sensations, and responses to different somatic practices.

You might ask yourself questions like, *"What sensations did I notice in my body today?"* or *"How did my emotional state shift during my practice?"* These kinds of reflections invite awareness rather than judgment. The goal is to stay curious and open to what your body and emotions are teaching you.

Here are examples of guided somatic questions you can ask yourself during the journaling process.

- *What physical sensations am I experiencing right now?*

____

____

____

____

____

- *Where in my body do I feel tension or discomfort?*

____

____

____

____

- *When I think about my current emotions, how do they manifest physically?*

- *Can I trace the journey of my breath—where does it feel most free, and where does it feel restricted?*

- *What images or memories arise when I focus on a specific part of my body?*

- *How does my posture reflect my current state of mind?*

- *What would it feel like to release the tension I'm holding in my body?*

- *How do certain thoughts or memories impact the way my body feels?*

- *What do I notice in my body when I focus on gratitude or joy?*

____

____

____

____

____

____

- *How does my body respond to the concept of change or uncertainty?*

____

____

____

____

____

Regularly engaging with these questions can help you recognize patterns, track emotional shifts, and strengthen your connection to your body's signals. Remember, the intention is to heighten your awareness. Each entry brings greater insight into your unique experience and supports your ongoing journey of embodied self-care.

Tracking Emotional and Physical Changes

Keeping a journal of your emotional and physical experiences can help you see just how much you're growing through your somatic practice. At first, noting brief reflections might feel simple or repetitive, but over time, patterns begin to surface. You may start to notice which practices consistently help you feel grounded or energized, and which ones reveal areas that need a little more care. These insights become a powerful guide, helping you make thoughtful adjustments to your self-care routine and deepening your understanding of what truly supports your well-being.

Example layout you can adapt:

Date	Physical Changes	Emotional Changes	Insights or Realizations	Overall Well-being
Keep track of when each reflection was noticed.	*Describe any physical changes, such as shifts in energy levels, sleep, or tension in your body.*	*Note any emotional shifts like mood, stress level, or a sense of calm.*	*Summarize anything meaningful you noticed while reflecting.*	*Rate how balanced or grounded you felt that day.*

To make the most of your journaling practice, try building a simple routine around it. You might set aside a few minutes at the same time each day or write after somatic exercises that feel especially meaningful. Journaling doesn't have to take long; short, consistent reflections often have the greatest impact. What matters most is showing up regularly. This simple habit keeps you connected to your progress and strengthens your commitment to personal growth and self-care.

Somatic Experiences for Improved Self-Care

True self-care goes beyond simply setting aside time to rest; it's about nurturing your whole self, body and mind. Somatic practices support this process by calming the nervous system, easing stress, and creating emotional balance. In this section, we'll explore a variety of approaches you can try, from gentle solo practices to group activities you can share with friends or family. Think of it as discovering new ways to move, connect, and restore your energy in everyday life.

Sound Bathing

Sound bathing is a soothing practice that helps quiet the mind and relax the body through the use of sound frequencies that interact with your body's natural rhythm. Instruments such as crystal bowls, gongs, or tuning forks create gentle vibrations that ease stress, release tension, and restore a sense of harmony throughout your system.

Imagine settling into a cozy space where soft lighting and stillness invite you inward. As the first notes fill the air, the tones begin to ripple through you; vibrations that seem to reach beneath the surface, loosening what has been held too tightly. The sound surrounds and moves through you, inviting your breath to deepen and your body to let go.

You may notice sensations shifting; warmth spreading, thoughts quieting, or emotions softening as each tone passes. Some sounds may feel grounding, others expansive, like waves gently carrying you back to center. Simply allow yourself to be present, letting the sound move where it's needed.

When the vibrations fade into silence, stay for a moment in that quiet. Feel the stillness they've left behind; a sense of spacious calm that lingers in both body and mind. Each session becomes a gentle reset, reminding you of your body's innate ability to release, restore, and return to balance.

Drawing Emotions

Creative expression can become a bridge between what you feel and what you understand about yourself. When emotions are too complex to name, art offers a gentle way to let them surface. Through color, line, and movement on a page, you can begin to see your inner world reflected back to you.

Next time you feel emotions stirring beneath the surface, gather a few simple supplies: colored pencils, crayons, or paints, and create a small space where you can work without distractions. Before you begin, pause for a moment. Take a few slow breaths and notice how you're feeling right now. Then, let your hand begin to move freely. Allow color to meet paper in whatever form it wishes: streaks, swirls, shapes, or patterns. There is no goal to reach, no image to perfect. This is an act of release and discovery rather than creation for display.

As you draw, stay present to what unfolds. You may notice a shift in your breathing, a softening of emotion, or perhaps an image emerging that surprises you. When you pause to look at what you've made, take it in gently. What colors stand out? What emotion do they seem to carry? Sometimes the act of looking reveals what the heart has been trying to say.

You might start to see familiar colors or shapes returning, small signatures of your emotional landscape. These patterns can become signposts, helping you recognize what your body and heart need as you continue your journey toward balance and self-understanding.

Laughter Yoga

Laughter yoga offers a joyful way to restore balance and lift your spirits. Blending mindful breathing with playful laughter helps to release tension, boost energy, and invite a sense of lightness into both body and mind. The focus isn't on humor or jokes, it's on the healing power of laughter itself. Even simulated laughter can awaken the same feel-good chemistry in the body, releasing endorphins that calm stress and create connection.

You can begin by standing or sitting comfortably, taking a few slow breaths to loosen your body. Allow a soft chuckle to rise, even if it feels a little forced at first. With each exhale, let the laughter grow;

short bursts, then deeper giggles, until it becomes natural and free-flowing. When practiced with others, laughter has a way of spreading easily. Eye contact, clapping, or playful gestures can spark genuine, contagious laughter that soon fills the space with warmth and energy.

Between moments of laughter, pause to breathe deeply and notice how you feel. Often, after the laughter subsides, a calm stillness remains; a quiet joy that lingers beneath the surface. Laughter yoga reminds us how healing it is to let go of self-consciousness, to be fully present, and to allow joy to rise through the simple act of laughter itself.

Key Takeaways

- Incorporating somatic exercises into your daily self-care routines is not about a one-size-fits-all solution; it's about discovering what works uniquely for you. Integrating these practices involves recognizing your daily needs and selecting approaches that resonate with both your emotional and physical needs
- This personalization empowers you to embrace an open and flexible mind as you learn to adapt and evolve your plans over time. By setting realistic goals and celebrating small milestones, the process becomes more sustainable, promoting long-term commitment.

In the end, creating a self-care routine that truly supports you is about staying curious and flexible. Keep exploring, adjusting, and allowing your practices to grow alongside you. What serves you now may shift as you continue to evolve, and that's part of the wisdom of self-care itself.

As we move forward, the focus turns inward toward the deeper roots of healing. The next chapter explores how family dynamics and inherited patterns can shape not only your emotional landscape but also the way your body holds and releases what it has carried through generations.

08.

Addressing Family Dynamics and Inherited Trauma

Out of suffering have emerged the strongest souls; the most massive characters are seared with scars. –Khalil Gibran

"

Your family operates like a living organism, with each member playing their role in the collective narrative. These stories have been told and retold from generation to generation, often embedding behaviors and emotional responses deep within your family's psyche.

Sometimes, these family stories carry unspoken traumas that ripple through generations, shaping behaviors, emotions, and even physical sensations. Your body often becomes the keeper of these untold experiences, storing them as tension, chronic pain, or unexplained discomfort; echoes of what those before you carried. Recognizing this connection between mind, body, and family history invites a deeper understanding of how your own healing is intertwined with the generations that came before you.

In this chapter, you'll explore how your body carries traces of the stories passed down through your family line. By bringing awareness to these inherited patterns, you begin to see how history lives within you, through emotions, reactions, and even physical sensations. Together, we'll look at ways to recognize and gently unravel these intergenerational threads, creating space for healing, understanding, and renewal.

Understanding Generational Trauma's Impact on the Body

Generational trauma is often an unseen inheritance, an emotional and physiological imprint passed down through families. The unprocessed pain of earlier generations can subtly shape how later ones respond to stress, express emotions, and form relationships.

A grandparent's unresolved grief or fear, for instance, may evolve into a parent's emotional restraint, eventually showing up in a child as anxiety, tension, or self-doubt. These patterns are carried not only in behavior but also in the body, influencing posture, breath, and nervous system responses. Recognizing these connections allows you to begin untangling the threads of inherited pain and create the possibility of healing within yourself and your lineage.

Identifying Body Responses to Inherited Trauma

The effects of generational trauma often show up in your own body, even when the original pain has long been buried. The weight of what earlier generations endured can surface as chronic tension, fatigue, or unexplained aches, signals of emotional stories that were never fully expressed. When the body cannot speak its distress, it holds it instead, carrying these unspoken narratives in muscle, breath, and posture. These sensations are not random; they are messages asking to be seen and understood so healing can begin.

You may also notice repeating emotional themes within your family, patterns of anxiety, depression, or self-protection that seem to echo through generations. Reflective practices can help you pause and ask, *Is this reaction truly mine, or does it belong to the past?* Exploring these questions brings powerful insight. It allows you to witness inherited behaviors with compassion, loosening their hold and making space for a new, more conscious way of being.

The following body awareness activity is designed to help you recognize trauma-related sensations in your body and uncover patterns or themes that may have been carried through your family line.

Instructions

1. Take a few deep breaths, inhaling through your nose and exhaling through your mouth. Allow your breath to anchor you in the present moment, noticing the rhythm and depth of each inhale and exhale.

2. Begin a thorough body scan from your head to your toes. Notice any areas of tension, discomfort, or sensations. Acknowledge what you feel without judgment, allowing yourself to become aware of these physical manifestations of your emotional experiences.

3. As you scan, contemplate any physical sensations that might connect to past trauma. Common symptoms may include notable tightness in the chest, a knot in the stomach, or oppressive feelings of heaviness. Seek to understand how these align with your emotional responses.

4. After the body scan, take a moment to explore your family history. Reflect on stories, behaviors, or challenges that may correlate with the sensations you identified. Consider questions like:

    a. *What recurring themes persist in your family's narrative?*

    b. *Are there specific coping mechanisms or behavioral patterns that appear to be passed down through generations?*

    c. *How do these patterns inform or exacerbate the physical symptoms you experience?*

5. Finally, take a few moments to ground yourself back in the present. Refocus on your breathing, and when you're ready, gently open your eyes, returning to your surroundings with a newfound sense of clarity regarding your experience and its connections to your family's history.

6. Reflect on your observations, feelings, and any patterns you've noticed. This process can help crystallize your understanding and provide a visual representation of your insights, linking the physical and emotional aspects of your experiences.

Awareness serves as a catalyst for breaking the cycle of inherited trauma. When you begin to recognize that certain behaviors, emotions, or physical discomforts may not have started with you, something shifts. This realization brings relief from self-blame and opens the way to understanding. Through this awareness, you develop deeper compassion, for yourself and for those who came before you. Healing begins here: in recognizing what has been passed down and what is truly yours to transform.

Healing Generational Trauma

Healing generational trauma starts with awareness, but real change happens through action. Once you begin to see the patterns that have been passed down, you can start choosing differently. This work doesn't happen in isolation; it often extends into your relationships and family.

Sometimes this means having honest conversations, setting new boundaries, or simply showing up with more compassion and patience. Little by little, these choices create space for new ways of connecting; ones built on understanding rather than pain. As each person begins to heal, the ripple effect can touch the whole family.

The following group exercise invites you to begin exploring generational healing with your family. Remember, uncovering and processing deep emotional wounds takes time; each person will move at their own pace, and that's completely okay. Approach the experience with patience, openness, and care for one another. If you find that strong emotions arise or you need extra support along the way, consider working with a family therapist who can guide you through the process safely.

Duration: 2–3 hours

Materials Needed

- comfortable seating arrangement
- journals and pens for each participant
- art supplies (colored pencils, markers, paper, etc.) for creative expression
- a timer for each discussion segment

Steps

1. **Creating a safe space (15 minutes):** Begin with a short opening circle. Invite each family member to share one positive word that represents their hopes for the session. Establish ground rules such as confidentiality, respect, and the importance of listening without interrupting.
2. **Guided discussion on generational trauma (30 minutes):** Choose a theme related to generational trauma (e.g., loss, abandonment, anxiety). Use open-ended questions to promote discussion, such as:
    a. *What emotions do you associate with this theme?*
    b. *Can you identify any experiences from our family history that relate to this?*
3. **Reflective listening (15 minutes):** Break into pairs for reflective listening. Each person takes turns sharing their

thoughts for 5 minutes while the partner listens without responding. After 5 minutes, the listener summarizes what they heard, allowing the speaker to clarify or expand on their feelings.

4. **Creative expression (30 minutes):** Provide art supplies and invite family members to create a piece that represents their feelings about the theme of generational trauma and healing. Encourage them to use colors, symbols, or phrases that resonate with their experiences.
5. **Sharing creative works (30 minutes):** Invite participants to share their artwork with the group. They can explain what it represents and how it connects to their feelings about generational trauma. Ensure a supportive environment where everyone feels comfortable sharing.
6. **Reflections and closing (30 minutes):** Come back together as a group and share reflections. Use prompts such as:
    a. *What did you learn about yourself or others?*
    b. *How can we support each other moving forward?*

End with a closing circle where everyone expresses one word or phrase that summarizes their feelings about the process. Acknowledge the courage it takes to engage in this work.

In essence, healing family dynamics and inherited trauma isn't something that can be solved quickly or neatly. It's about understanding how the past, present, and future are all woven together within your family story.

Every moment of tension, every feeling of love, and even every breath of relief may carry echoes from generations before you. And yet, within these connections lies immense potential; the opportunity to rewrite old patterns and create a new legacy built on awareness, compassion, and understanding.

Exploring Family Therapy Techniques

Family therapy often draws on *family systems theory*, developed by psychiatrist Dr. Murray Bowen. This approach helps you understand how family dynamics shape individual thoughts, emotions, and behaviors (Cohen, 2023). It suggests that patterns of communication, emotional responses, and belief systems can be unconsciously repeated across generations, influencing how family members relate to one another and navigate conflict.

You can think of your family as an interconnected system; when one person changes, the entire system shifts in response. For example, if you were raised in an environment where emotions were minimized, you might find it difficult to express vulnerability in adulthood.

In the following section, we'll explore somatic-based techniques that help families work through these inherited patterns, addressing issues such as enmeshment, blurred boundaries, and the lingering effects of generational trauma.

Unlearning Invalidation and Apathy

A key aspect of addressing trauma within families lies in the process of validation. Validation means recognizing and acknowledging a person's feelings or experiences without necessarily agreeing with them. It involves showing respect for someone else's perspective, even if your own views differ.

For example, you might not share the same feelings about what happened during a family event, but it's important to listen when a sibling expresses how that event affected them. This kind of support helps create an environment where feelings can be openly shared, leading to better understanding among family members.

Emotional validation helps build trust within a family. When one member shares their feelings or experiences and feels heard, they are more likely to share again in the future. This exchange creates a safety net where vulnerability is met with understanding rather than judgment.

Beyond invalidation, some family members may experience emotional numbness or indifference toward one another. This sense of *apathy* often develops when people feel overwhelmed, disconnected, or emotionally exhausted. When this happens, it can be hard to show empathy or respond with care, leading to emotional distance within the family.

To begin rebuilding connection, try setting aside regular, distraction-free time together. Shared activities, like cooking a meal, walking, or playing a game, can help ease tension and restore a sense of closeness. When the family feels more relaxed and connected, deeper conversations and emotional openness tend to follow naturally.

Below is a simple family activity designed to encourage validation, connection, and shared experiences that open the door to meaningful conversation.

Instructions

1. Gather your family in a cozy spot and sit in a circle.
2. Each member will take turns sharing a story from their life. It can be a funny, memorable, or even a challenging experience.
3. You could set a timer for 3–5 minutes per person to keep things flowing.
4. After each story, family members will respond with affirmations and supportive comments to validate feelings and experiences.
5. Encourage each person to ask follow-up questions to deepen the discussion.

Here are conversation prompts you can use to start discussions:

- *How did that experience make you feel at the time?*
- *What did you learn from that situation?*
- *Can you relate to that experience in any way?*
- *What would you have done differently, if anything?*
- *How did that story shape who you are today?*
- *Is there a moment from that story that stands out the most to you?*
- *How can we support each other in similar situations moving forward?*

The purpose of this exercise is to create space where every voice can be heard and valued. When family members practice listening with empathy and responding with kindness, old patterns of invalidation begin to shift. As this simple act of sharing and validating one another becomes more familiar, it can rebuild trust, strengthen bonds, and nurture an atmosphere of emotional safety where healing naturally unfolds.

Techniques for Family Engagement

Moving into more practical approaches, communication exercises can help strengthen family bonds. These include practices like active listening and structured dialogues, where each person has the chance to speak without interruption. Such activities encourage genuine understanding and help family members build deeper empathy for one another.

Family engagement naturally changes over time, shifting with the different seasons of life. It may feel easy to stay connected when children are still at home, yet more challenging once they leave for college or begin their own lives. Major transitions, new responsibilities, and unexpected challenges can all influence how closely family members stay in touch and how they show up for one another.

The following activity is designed to help strengthen family engagement during times when connection feels distant. Follow the steps and invite your family members to take part with an open mind and a willingness to reconnect.

Instructions

1. Begin by inviting each family member to think of a positive family value or personal strength—for example, kindness, honesty, teamwork, or patience.
2. Sit together in a circle or cozy space where everyone can see and hear each other. Explain the purpose of this activity: to express and celebrate your family's values through a fun, lighthearted round of charades.
3. Take turns choosing a value to act out silently for about a minute, while the rest of the family tries to guess what it

is. Encourage creativity and laughter—there's no need for perfection.

4. After each round, pause to reflect together. Talk about what that value means to each person and how it shows up in everyday life. You might ask, "*When have we shown this value recently?*" or "*How can we practice it more often?*"
5. Continue until everyone has had a turn, or until you've explored several values that feel meaningful to your family.
6. End the activity by reflecting on how these values can strengthen family bonds and how they can be incorporated into daily activities.

Keep a lighthearted approach, encouraging laughter and playful interaction. Emphasize the importance of listening to each other's perspectives during discussions.

Building family engagement takes intention, but it doesn't have to be complicated. Simple moments of laughter, shared values, and honest communication can do more to strengthen connection than grand gestures ever could. What matters most is showing up, listening, participating, and staying open to each other's perspectives. These small acts of engagement nurture a sense of belonging and remind everyone that family connection, no matter how it shifts, can always be renewed.

Reconciling Family Conflict

Conflict within families is inevitable, but incorporating somatic awareness into the process can turn tense moments into opportunities for healing. Simple practices like mindful breathing or grounding exercises can help everyone stay centered and calm, even when emotions run high. By pausing to take a few deep breaths before responding, you give your body a chance to settle and your mind the clarity to communicate with compassion and understanding.

The following exercise is designed to help you prepare for conversations involving family conflict or sensitive topics while staying calm, centered, and mindful throughout the discussion.

1. **Set the intention:** What positive intention will you set for this discussion? Write down your reflection on what you hope to achieve.

2. **Practice active listening:** Describe a situation where a family member expressed something important to them. How will you focus on their perspective and acknowledge their feelings? Note down the phrases you can use.

3. **Use "I" statements:** Identify a feeling you want to express. Frame your statement using "I." For example: "I feel _when _."

4. **Take breaks if necessary:** Recall a time when emotions escalated during a conversation. How did you handle it? Write down a suggestion for taking a break.

____

____

____

____

____

____

5. **Practice mindfulness techniques:** What mindfulness technique do you plan to use during the discussion? Describe how you will implement it.

____

____

____

____

____

____

____

6. **Find common ground:** After discussing differing viewpoints, what shared values or goals do you hope to embody? How can you ensure the conversation steers in this direction?

7. **Agree to disagree:** Write a reflection on how you can show mutual respect when having differing opinions. What strategies will you use?

8. **Follow-up:** How will you check in with each other after the discussion? Write down your plan to express appreciation and acknowledge progress made.

Conflict is a natural part of family life, and the way it's handled can shape the strength of your relationships. Approaching difficult conversations with mindfulness and body awareness helps create space for understanding and emotional safety. Each time you pause to breathe, listen, and speak with intention, you reinforce trust and compassion within your family.

Somatic Exercises to Heal Inherited Trauma

When working to heal inherited trauma within the family, somatic practices can help restore connection and create a sense of unity. These approaches focus on strengthening emotional bonds and releasing stored tension or emotions that may have been carried across generations. The following exercises offer practical ways to deepen awareness, encourage empathy, and support healing within your family system.

Family Tree Visualization

Family tree visualization is a meaningful exercise that helps you explore the emotional connections within your family system. By visually mapping your family tree, you can begin to notice patterns, relationships, and feelings that surface as you reflect on each connection. This practice invites you to consider how past interactions and generational ties continue to shape the dynamics you experience today.

As you work through this visualization, you may start to notice subtle patterns and emotional threads that have shaped your family's behavior over time. These insights can reveal how inherited experiences or unresolved trauma continue to influence your own life and relationships. Developing this kind of awareness is an important step toward creating change, both within yourself and within your family.

Instructions

1. Take a quiet moment to visualize your family tree, not just by names, but by emotional connections.
2. Begin by imagining yourself at the center. Around you, picture your closest family members: parents, siblings, grandparents, or others who played a meaningful role.
3. As you bring each person to mind, notice what emotions or sensations arise. You might associate warm feelings with some, tension or confusion with others. Think of colors that could represent those emotions: green for comfort, red for conflict, yellow for mixed or changing feelings.
4. Reflect on the nature of these relationships. What moments or memories stand out? Which patterns or traits seem to repeat through generations?
5. As you notice these themes, try to connect them.
6. Take a few slow breaths and sit with your visualization. Consider what you've discovered about your family patterns and how they influence your current relationships.
7. Ask yourself:
    - *Which connections feel nourishing?*
    - *Which might still need healing or clearer boundaries?*
    - *What insights or emotions stand out most right now?*

If comfortable, share your visualization with trusted family members. This can open up discussions about family dynamics and lead to greater understanding and healing.

As you finish your family tree visualization, take a moment to reflect on what you've uncovered. Approach your insights with curiosity and compassion, allowing them to deepen your understanding of the connections within your family. The patterns you notice can offer a valuable perspective, helping you make conscious choices that lead to healthier relationships and emotional balance. Awareness becomes a bridge between understanding the past and creating a more grounded, connected future.

Family Dialogue Role Play

Family dialogue role play is a helpful way to explore and improve family dynamics. In this exercise, family members reenact conversations or common situations to better understand one another's perspectives. Stepping into someone else's role can build empathy and reveal what each person may be feeling beneath their words. Practicing this kind of open communication in a safe, supportive setting helps uncover unspoken tensions and encourages healthier, more compassionate ways of relating.

This exercise helps strengthen empathy and encourages you and your family members to express yourselves with greater authenticity. Through this practice, you can begin to create a more supportive and emotionally balanced family environment. Follow the steps below to get started.

Steps

1. Begin by selecting a situation that allows for different perspectives, such as planning a family vacation, deciding on a family meal, or discussing boundaries.
2. Each family member should take on a specific role relevant to the scenario. For example, in a vacation planning scenario, roles could include the Organizer, the Budget-Conscious Member, the Adventurer, and the Relaxation Seeker.
3. Create a comfortable environment to engage in this role play. You can use props or set up areas that resemble the scenario to make it more immersive.

4. Each family member should express their character's thoughts, feelings, and opinions related to the scenario. Encourage them to explain the reasoning behind their character's views.
5. While one member is speaking, others should listen without interrupting. After each perspective, family members can ask clarifying questions to better understand their viewpoints.
6. After all perspectives have been shared, have a discussion about how each family member feels about their character's perspective and the perspectives of others.
7. Work together to find solutions or compromises that take into account everyone's feelings and perspectives. This promotes collaboration and understanding.
8. After the activity, spend a few minutes reflecting as a family on what was learned about accepting and expressing different perspectives and feelings.

Family dialogue role play works best when everyone stays open to exploration and listens with genuine interest. The goal is to notice how each person expresses themselves and responds to others. With continued practice, conversations can begin to feel more natural, and moments of tension can transform into opportunities for connection and growth. This simple exercise can remind families that meaningful change often begins with a willingness to listen and engage with sincerity.

Grounding Through Rituals

Creating simple rituals can be a meaningful way to honor your family history and feel connected to your roots. A ritual is any intentional act performed with awareness; it gives space to pause, reflect, and reconnect with what matters most. It's a gentle reminder of connection, both to your family and to yourself. Each moment of reflection strengthens your sense of belonging and continuity, linking past and present through simple, mindful action. This small practice can become an anchor, grounding you in peace, gratitude, and the enduring presence of those who came before you.

If you're interested in creating your own rituals, follow these guidelines:

1. Discuss what values and beliefs are important to your family, such as love, gratitude, or togetherness.
2. Ensure that all family members have a say in creating rituals. This fosters a sense of ownership and commitment.
3. Look at existing family traditions or cultural practices that resonate with your family.
4. Decide how often you want to engage in these rituals—daily, weekly, monthly, or seasonally.
5. Select specific activities that everyone enjoys and that align with your family values, such as game nights, storytelling sessions, or outdoor adventures.
6. Incorporate symbols or items that represent your family's identity, like a special dish, a family motto, or a unique gesture.
7. Regularly assess the significance and enjoyment of the rituals and make adjustments to ensure they remain meaningful for everyone involved.

Family rituals hold meaning beyond the actions themselves. They nurture connection, belonging, and a sense of continuity across generations. When created with intention, these shared practices remind each person that they are part of something enduring and significant, and become sources of comfort and unity, strengthening the values that keep your family close.

Key Takeaways

- Recognizing that your body often holds onto the stories and tensions passed down from prior generations marks the first step toward healing. By examining physical, emotional, and behavioral patterns, you can begin to untangle the threads linking past traumas to your current behaviors.
- Throughout this chapter, you have been encouraged to reflect on whether your reactions are truly your own or echoes resonating from your familial history. Uncovering this distinction allows you to approach healing with empathy, embracing both self-awareness and compassion for those who came before you.
- Reflective practices like mindfulness, journaling, and somatic exercises assist in navigating these inherited challenges. They serve as tools for bringing unresolved issues to light, encouraging introspection, and breaking repetitive cycles. Through such practices, you learn to release physical tensions and rewrite narratives that no longer serve you.

Healing is rarely a solitary path; it unfolds within the connections we share. Inviting your family into open, heartfelt dialogue creates opportunities for understanding and growth that extend beyond individual change. As you move forward, let the insights you've gained guide your actions and deepen the bonds you share with those closest to you.

In the next chapter, we'll explore somatic practices designed to strengthen emotional resilience, helping you stay grounded, balanced, and connected as you continue your healing journey.

09.

Developing Emotional Resilience

You are the sky. Everything else—it's just the weather. –Pema Chödrön

"

Developing emotional resilience is an ongoing journey that grows through self-awareness and adaptability. It helps you meet life's challenges with steadiness and confidence, even during times of uncertainty. Resilience involves staying present with your emotions, understanding what they're communicating, and responding in ways that support your overall well-being.

In this chapter, you'll explore somatic strategies that strengthen your emotional foundation and expand your capacity to recover from stress. Through these practices, you can build greater balance, confidence, and a deeper sense of trust in yourself as you navigate the changing landscapes of life.

Identifying and Building on Emotional Strengths

Recognizing your emotional strengths helps you understand how they shape your thoughts, behaviors, and relationships. This awareness allows you to draw on those strengths more intentionally, especially during times of challenge or change. In this section, you'll learn how to identify the qualities that support your resilience and use them as a steady foundation for continued growth and emotional balance.

Strengths Inventory List

Recognizing your inherent emotional strengths is an essential part of building resilience. These qualities are unique to you, much like a fingerprint, and acknowledging them strengthens your sense of self-efficacy while deepening your understanding of who you are.

Emotional strengths can take many forms, such as empathy, patience, creativity, optimism, or the ability to remain calm under pressure. When you identify and reflect on these qualities, you begin to see how they influence your choices, relationships, and responses to life's challenges.

To help you uncover and build upon these strengths, the following guided reflection will guide you through a simple self-assessment designed to highlight the traits that support your emotional well-being.

Instructions

Go through the following questions, reflecting on times in the past when you have displayed these emotional strengths, and what might have been the motivation.

Questions

1. **Resilience:** Think of a time when you faced a significant challenge and managed to overcome it. What specific emotions did you feel during that time? How did you cope with the situation, and what strengths did you rely on to bounce back?

____

____

____

____

____

2. **Empathy:** Reflect on an experience where you helped someone in need. What emotions did you share with them, and how did it affect your relationship? Which qualities within yourself did you draw upon to provide support?

3. **Courage:** Recall a moment when you took a risk or stepped out of your comfort zone. What motivated you to act despite fear or uncertainty? What inner strengths did you discover or develop as a result of that experience?

4. **Adaptability:** Think back to a time when you had to adjust your plans or expectations unexpectedly. How did you handle the change? What strategies did you use to adapt, and which strengths did you uncover about yourself through that experience?

5. **Gratitude:** Identify a situation where you felt an overwhelming sense of gratitude. What key moments or actions led you to that feeling? How does acknowledging that strength of gratitude impact your perspective on life?

6. **Optimism:** Reflect on a challenging time when you maintained a positive outlook. What thoughts or self-talk helped you stay optimistic? What do you believe about yourself that fueled this sense of hope?

7. **Creativity:** Recall a moment when you found a unique solution to a problem. What motivated your creative thinking, and what emotions accompanied that process? How did this experience reveal your strengths in innovation?

8. **Connection:** Think about a relationship that significantly uplifted you. How have the feelings of love and support from that relationship shaped your sense of self? What strengths did you rely on to nurture that connection?

9. **Mindfulness:** Reflect on an experience where you were fully present and aware. What practices or activities help you achieve this state? How has mindfulness revealed your emotional strengths during difficult moments?

10. **Self-acceptance:** Consider a time when you embraced your true self despite outside judgment. What emotions did you experience during that moment of acceptance? What strengths did you recognize in yourself that contributed to your personal growth?

Taking time to identify your emotional strengths helps you recognize the inner resources that have carried you through life's challenges. These qualities are already within you, waiting to be acknowledged and nurtured.

As you continue to reflect, notice how each strength supports your growth, confidence, and ability to recover from stress. Building awareness of these traits not only enhances resilience but also deepens your trust in yourself and your capacity to navigate whatever life brings.

Storytelling for Building Emotional Strength

Personal stories of recovery remind us what resilience looks like in real life. Through these narratives, you can see how emotional strengths support healing and growth. Reading about someone who faced the loss of a job, a relationship, or another life challenge with perseverance and adaptability can spark insight and encouragement for your own journey. These stories provide more than inspiration; they offer guidance on how to draw upon your own strengths when life feels uncertain.

If you struggle with unforgiveness, hearing from individuals who have turned their empathy into a bridge for rebuilding connections provides a vivid illustration of emotional strengths at work. These stories emphasize the potential within you to rise above difficulties with confidence and determination.

The following activity will help you find inspiration in the triumphs of those around you.

Instructions

1. Choose celebrities or local community members who have overcome significant challenges. Research their backgrounds and experiences.
2. Source five key elements from their stories:
    a. *What specific adversity or obstacle did the individual confront?*
    b. *What moment or event changed their trajectory or mindset?*
    c. *Who supported them through their journey (friends, family, mentors)?*
    d. *What insights or lessons have they shared as a result of their experiences?*

e. *What successes or accomplishments have they achieved after overcoming their challenges?*

3. Take the gathered information and reshape the inspirational story from the individual's perspective, reflecting their thoughts, feelings, and the lessons they've learned along the way.

____

____

____

____

____

____

____

As you explore these stories, notice the common thread that runs through them, the courage to keep going and the willingness to grow through pain. Each story is a reminder that strength is not the absence of struggle but the ability to transform it into wisdom. When you connect with these narratives, you're also reconnecting with your own capacity for resilience, compassion, and hope.

Movement-Based Emotions Activation

Incorporating movement-based exercises specifically designed to target emotional strengths helps ensure that these qualities remain accessible and robust. For instance, a simple daily stretching routine can promote flexibility—not just physically, but emotionally, enabling you to adapt more easily to change. Additionally, mindful walking meditations encourage introspection, enhance self-awareness, and reinforce self-acceptance as key components of resilience.

Here is a movement-based emotions activation exercise called "Emotion Flow" that consists of distinct phases that target specific positive emotions through various body motions. Make sure you have enough floor space to carry out the movements below.

Movements

1. **Joyful jumps:** Start with a series of small, energetic jumps while smiling broadly. As you jump, envision joy radiating from your heart, filling your entire body. Focus on the buoyant feeling in your legs and let it uplift your spirit.
2. **Gratitude waves:** Stand tall and extend your arms wide, then slowly sweep them down and back up while taking deep breaths. As you move, think of three things you are grateful for, letting each wave signify your appreciation for those aspects of your life.
3. **Calm sway:** Shift your weight from side to side in a gentle sway, closing your eyes if comfortable. Focus on calming your mind, letting your body follow the rhythm of your breath. Visualize a peaceful place that brings you tranquility, fostering feelings of serenity.
4. **Confidence stance:** Stand in a strong power pose with your hands on your hips. Take deep breaths, and with each inhalation, imagine your confidence growing. Hold this position for a few moments to cultivate and amplify your self-assurance.
5. **Release and reflect:** End the exercise with slow, fluid arm movements that mimic the act of letting go. As your arms move, think of any negative emotions or worries dissolving. Once complete, take a moment to reflect on the positive feelings you experienced throughout the exercise.

As you practice "Emotion Flow," notice how your mood shifts and your body responds. Each movement offers a way to reconnect with emotions that strengthen and sustain you. This mindful use of movement can become a trusted tool for grounding, renewal, and emotional balance; something you can return to whenever you need to realign your energy and remember your inner resilience.

Ultimately, building emotional resilience is a lifelong journey of self-discovery and growth. When you take time to recognize and nurture your strengths, you create a steady foundation for meeting life's challenges with confidence. The stories of others remind us that resilience lives in all of us, while somatic practices give us tangible ways to strengthen it each day. Together, they form a path of healing, one built on awareness, compassion, and the power of returning to yourself.

Creating Space for Emotional Expression

Emotional expression is the ability, and the courage, to share what you truly feel. As we move through life, this often becomes harder. Self-consciousness, past hurt, or fear of judgment can make us hold back what needs to be voiced. But the good news is that emotional openness can be relearned. Through gentle practice, we can train ourselves to communicate with both honesty and compassion, building emotional resilience along the way.

The following somatic exercises are designed to help you reconnect with your emotions, express them safely, and build confidence in sharing your inner world.

Vulnerability Training Exercise

Emotions are deeply intertwined with your physical and mental health. When you suppress them, they often manifest physically as tension, headaches, or even chronic pain. The act of bottling up emotions can lead to increased stress levels, contributing to various health problems over time. On the other hand, openly expressing emotions allows for a release that prevents these negative physical manifestations.

Acknowledging vulnerability as a strength rather than a weakness shifts your perspective on emotional openness. Sharing feelings, whether joy, sorrow, or frustration, connects you with others. This vulnerability strengthens relationships, transforming personal connections into sources of support rather than stress.

The following vulnerability exercise will help you learn to be more open in sharing your inner thoughts and feelings through exposure therapy. Before proceeding to the next level, check in with your body and assess your comfort levels.

Level 1: Private Reflection

Start by *taking time to reflect on a sensitive topic* that feels relevant to your current emotional landscape. You might think about a past experience or a situation that often brings up strong feelings. Notice what emotions or thoughts surface as you think about it.

Level 2: Sharing with Someone You Trust

When you feel ready, consider *talking about your reflections* with someone you feel safe and supported by. This could be a friend, partner, or mentor who listens with compassion. Focus on expressing how the experience feels for you rather than trying to "fix" it. Pay attention to how your body responds during and after sharing.

Level 3: Community Connection

As you gain confidence, the next step involves sharing your experiences in a small group setting. This could be a therapy group or a supportive circle of friends. Be prepared to discuss your thoughts and feelings again. For example, you could join a group focused on mental health where members take turns sharing similar experiences and feelings.

Level 4: Public Sharing

Finally, consider sharing your experiences publicly, whether through social media, a blog, or a public forum. This step can be daunting, but it allows for broader support and understanding. For instance, you might write a blog post about your journey with anxiety, explaining how it impacts you and encouraging others to open up about their struggles.

Remember to continuously check in with your body at each level, ensuring you are comfortable with the process. Taking these gradual steps can help you become more open in sharing your inner thoughts and feelings.

Emotional Release Through Artistic Expression

To facilitate safe emotional release, creative outlets can be incredibly beneficial. Engaging in art, dance, and writing provides tangible ways to express emotions without the need for words, offering a sense of relief and validation. For instance, painting or drawing can help articulate complex emotions through color and form, bypassing verbal limitations. Similarly, movement practices like dance or yoga encourage the release of stored tension and allow emotions to flow freely through your body, leading to a more integrated sense of self.

The following reflection invites you to explore artistic or creative ways to express emotions and restore calm in your body. You may choose one form or combine several that resonate with you. Whether through movement, music, color, or imagery, allow your creativity to guide you toward understanding your emotions and cultivating inner balance.

1. **Nature sculpting:** You can use natural materials like leaves, stones, or twigs to create small sculptures that represent your emotions. Arrange them in a way that expresses how you feel.
2. **Body mapping:** If you'd like, try lying down on a large sheet of paper and tracing your outline. Consider using colors, symbols, or patterns to fill in areas that represent different emotions you've experienced.
3. **Emotional mosaic:** Explore the idea of gathering small items (such as buttons, fabric scraps, or beads) that resonate with different emotions, and use them to create a mosaic art piece symbolizing how you feel.
4. **Personal aroma creation:** Experiment with blending essential oils or natural scents that evoke certain emotions and create a unique fragrance. Reflect on the emotions each scent represents for you.
5. **Mood food art:** Play with expressing your emotions through food. Prepare a meal or snack that mirrors your mood through color and texture, and take a moment to appreciate the artistic side before enjoying it.
6. **Movement journaling:** Give yourself permission to move freely in response to your emotions, as if you're dancing without rules or rhythm. Afterward, take a quiet moment to reflect on what the movement revealed.
7. **Emotional quilt:** If you'd like, create a small quilt or fabric collage that represents various emotions you've felt. Use different fabrics, patterns, or stitches to denote unique feelings.

Each form of creative expression gives emotion a safe place to land. Whether through color, movement, scent, or sound, you're allowing your inner world to take shape in a way words often can't. The goal is to feel something shift inside you. As you practice expressing emotion through art and movement, you'll begin to notice a deeper calm, a sense of release, and a growing trust in your body's natural capacity to heal through creation.

Identifying Emotionally Safe People

Having safe, supportive people around you makes emotional growth so much easier. These are the relationships where you can show up as your full self, where your feelings are heard, respected, and met with empathy instead of judgment. When you find people who value openness and genuine connection, you begin to feel seen and accepted in a way that allows healing to unfold naturally.

This kind of safety can exist in many places, within your family, close friendships, or in supportive communities and groups. Surrounding yourself with people who listen and understand creates an environment where vulnerability becomes strength. These relationships don't just help you feel safe; they remind you that you don't have to navigate life's challenges alone.

Below is a checklist that you can go through to assess whether you have found someone who is emotionally safe. If you answer yes to most of these questions, consider including them in your support network. Remember to continuously work on becoming an emotionally safe individual for them, too.

Question	Yes	No
1. Does this person listen to you without interrupting? *Listening without interruption indicates respect and a willingness to understand your feelings.*		
2. Do you feel comfortable expressing your thoughts and feelings around them? *A sense of comfort signifies that the person respects your emotions and vulnerabilities.*		

3. Does this person validate your feelings, acknowledging your emotions without judgment? *Validation shows that they recognize and accept your emotional experiences.*		
4. Is this person trustworthy, keeping your confidences private? *Trustworthiness is key for emotional safety: It reinforces that your shared experiences are secure.*		
5. Do they communicate openly and honestly with you? *Open communication creates an environment of transparency and trust.*		
6. Can you depend on this person to support you in difficult times? *Reliability in times of need demonstrates their commitment to your well-being.*		
7. Do they refrain from using manipulation or guilt to influence your decisions? *Avoiding manipulation indicates respect for your autonomy and decisions.*		
8. Do they encourage your personal growth and respect your boundaries? *Support for personal growth combined with respect for boundaries shows they care about your well-being.*		
9. Do they share their own vulnerabilities with you, promoting mutual trust? *Mutual sharing of vulnerabilities strengthens emotional connections and trust.*		
10. Have they reacted positively when you've expressed your needs or feelings? *Positive reactions indicate they are open and willing to engage with you emotionally.*		

As you reflect on your answers, remember that emotionally safe relationships develop through consistency, trust, and mutual care. They're built over time through shared honesty and the willingness to listen and grow together. The more you surround yourself with people who honor your truth, the more supported you'll feel in expressing it. Emotional safety isn't only something we find; it's something we nurture through presence, empathy, and respect.

Somatic Exercises to Get Comfortable With Difficult Emotions

In this section, we will explore exercises designed to help you connect with and process difficult emotions. Emotions can often feel overwhelming, and they tend to manifest physically within our bodies. By engaging in somatic practices, we can learn to tune into these sensations, acknowledge them, and release their grip on our well-being. These exercises will provide a gentle pathway for you to become more comfortable with your emotional experiences, transforming them from barriers into catalysts for growth and healing. Now, let's look into the specific somatic exercises that will aid in processing these challenging emotions.

Emotional Weather Report

Let's begin with the idea of visualizing your emotions as weather patterns. Imagine your emotions as ever-changing skies—sometimes clear and blue, other times stormy and overcast. This visualization helps create a sense of awareness and distance, allowing you to observe emotions without becoming overwhelmed by them.

Journaling can be an effective tool here. By writing down how you perceive these emotional 'weather changes,' you can reflect on patterns over time and understand how certain triggers affect your emotional state. Use your journal as a safe space to pour out your feelings, much like noting the day's forecast; this exercise trains you to acknowledge and anticipate your emotional climate.

Here's an example of how you could describe your daily emotional weather reflection:

Date	Emotional Weather	Description	Action Needed
YYYY-MM-DD	Sunny	Feeling energized and optimistic	Embrace positivity.
YYYY-MM-DD	Partly cloudy	Mild concerns or stress lingering	Take a break and breathe.
YYYY-MM-DD	Overcast	Feeling down or lethargic	Reach out for support.
YYYY-MM-DD	Thunderstorm	Experiencing anger or frustration	Reflect and find healthy outlets.
YYYY-MM-DD	Snowy	Sense of isolation or sadness	Connect with loved ones.
YYYY-MM-DD	Windy	Anxiety or restlessness making it hard to focus	Practice mindfulness.
YYYY-MM-DD	Foggy	Confusion or uncertainty about decisions	Clarify thoughts and priorities.
YYYY-MM-DD	Clear night sky	Peaceful and content with life	Celebrate small victories.

As you continue this practice, notice how your emotional weather shifts over time and what helps the storms pass more gently. This awareness doesn't stop difficult emotions from appearing, but it changes your relationship with them. Instead of being swept away, you learn to observe, understand, and respond with patience. Over time, your inner landscape begins to feel more balanced, anchored in awareness, yet open to change.

Somatic Soundscapes

Music has a remarkable way of reflecting what's happening inside us. It can stir memories, amplify joy, or bring comfort when words fall short. Creating playlists that match different emotions: joy, sadness, anger, calm, gives you a gentle way to express and move through what you're feeling.

When an emotion feels especially strong, let the music guide you. Play the song that matches your mood and allow your body to respond naturally. Maybe you dance, sway, or simply tap your foot to the rhythm. Movement helps the emotion find its way out, like shaking off raindrops after a sudden downpour.

Here is an example of a playlist that can boost your motivation when you're in a slump:

1. "Fight Song" by Rachel Platten
2. "Stronger" by Kelly Clarkson
3. "Can't Stop the Feeling!" by Justin Timberlake
4. "Good as Hell" by Lizzo
5. "Rise Up" by Andra Day
6. "Don't Stop Believin'" by Journey
7. "Eye of the Tiger" by Survivor
8. "Hall of Fame" by The Script ft. Will.i.am
9. "Shake It Off" by Taylor Swift
10. "Titanium" by Sia

As you explore your own soundscapes, notice how different rhythms, lyrics, and tones shift your mood and energy. Music can become a form of emotional dialogue between your body and your spirit, a reminder that healing doesn't always happen in stillness. Sometimes it happens in motion, through melody, and in the simple act of letting yourself feel fully alive.

Personal Mantras

Mantras can serve as powerful tools for you to process difficult emotions. By repeating a calming phrase or affirmation, you create a mental anchor that brings your focus back to the present moment. This practice can help to soothe overwhelming feelings, allowing you to confront and understand them in a more manageable way.

When you use personal mantras, you give yourself permission to experience your emotions without judgment. The repetitive nature of mantras can build a sense of stability and safety, which might be particularly comforting during turbulent times.

To craft personal mantras for processing difficult emotions, follow these steps:

1. Take a moment to reflect on the specific difficult emotion you are experiencing (e.g., anger, sadness, anxiety). Notice the emotion and any accompanying thoughts or feelings.

2. Recognize that it's okay to feel this way. Think of a short sentence that validates your feelings, such as *"It's okay to feel sad right now."*

3. Think of a phrase or affirmation that resonates with you and offers comfort. This could be something like *"I am safe," "I am enough,"* or *"This too shall pass."*

4. Create a personal mantra by combining your acknowledgment of the emotion with your calming phrase. For example, *"It's okay to feel sad; I am safe in this moment."*

5. Use the mantra during moments of distress. Repeat it aloud or in your mind to help center yourself and process your emotions.

---

6. After a few days, reflect on how the mantra has affected your emotional experience. Feel free to adjust or create new mantras as needed based on your evolving feelings.

Personal mantras remind you that comfort and strength can come from within. Each time you repeat your chosen words, you're reinforcing a sense of safety and self-trust, teaching your mind and body that they can return to calm even in moments of turmoil. These affirmations become more than phrases; they become companions on your healing journey, helping you meet your emotions with steadiness and compassion.

Key Takeaways

- Identifying and building on your emotional strengths can significantly bolster your emotional resilience. By recognizing qualities like empathy, patience, and creativity, you lay down a foundation for personal growth.
- Through reflection on past experiences, you're able to see how these strengths have supported you and how they can be further developed. This insight is crucial as it empowers you to construct a personal inventory of your emotional assets, transforming them into a resource that allows you to face adversity with confidence.
- In addition, integrating somatic exercises provides practical ways to connect your body and mind, enhancing your journey toward resilience. Practices such as movement-based exercises and artistic expression make these emotional qualities more accessible and ensure their robustness over time.

Embracing these somatic tools is an ongoing practice; a way of caring for your emotional well-being and staying connected to your own resilience. As you continue to integrate what you've learned, you'll notice how small moments of awareness can help you stay centered, even when life feels unpredictable.

In the next chapter, we'll look at some of the common challenges that can arise along the healing journey and explore practical ways to move through them with patience and self-understanding.

10.

Overcoming Barriers to Somatic Healing

What happens when people open their hearts? They get better. –Haruki Murakami

"

Overcoming barriers to somatic healing means dealing with a mix of societal views and personal experiences. This chapter looks at these issues and the challenges you might face. By understanding how cultural beliefs shape what people think about somatic practices, you can start to break down the stigma around this kind of therapy. These barriers aren't just outside; they are feelings you may also have within yourself, affecting how you approach your healing journey and how you see body-centered therapies as valid options.

Navigating Stigma and Misunderstanding Around Somatic Practices

For a long time, psychology has shaped how we think about mental health, emphasizing talk-based therapies over those that include the body's wisdom. As a result, approaches like somatic therapy have sometimes been misunderstood or dismissed as unconventional.

Society often views mind-centered methods, such as psychotherapy or counseling, as more credible or familiar, while body-focused practices are seen as alternative or experimental. But this perception overlooks how deeply the body and mind are connected, and how somatic awareness can open new doors to understanding, healing, and self-discovery.

Because of these long-standing cultural beliefs that prioritize the mind over the body, somatic work has often been misunderstood or minimized. For many people, this leads to feelings of doubt or hesitation, especially when others don't understand or accept body-centered approaches to healing. These misunderstandings can make you feel uncertain about exploring somatic therapy, even though the body has always been a vital part of emotional and psychological recovery.

Acknowledging this history helps you release any shame or self-consciousness you may feel about pursuing this kind of therapy. The more you understand where these biases come from, the more empowered you become to trust your own experience and embrace what truly supports your healing.

Reframing Conversations About Somatic Therapy

If you feel drawn to somatic therapy, take time to learn about it from reliable sources rather than relying solely on others' opinions or misconceptions. Explore what the process involves and how it can help release the emotions and tension the body often holds onto after trauma or prolonged stress. Understanding the principles behind it allows you to make an informed choice based on curiosity and self-awareness rather than fear or uncertainty.

If, after exploring it, somatic therapy resonates with you, consider sharing what you've learned with others. Speaking openly about your experience can help demystify body-centered healing and encourage more compassionate conversations around alternative therapies. Advocacy doesn't mean convincing others, it simply means giving voice to your truth and helping create understanding where there may once have been doubt.

Having community support is equally important. The journey to understanding and normalizing somatic therapy doesn't have to happen in isolation. Joining holistic or wellness groups can offer the sense of belonging and encouragement that makes the process feel lighter and more sustainable.

Within these communities, you'll find others who value embodied healing and are eager to share their stories, insights, and experiences. Together, you create a supportive space where somatic practices are not only validated but celebrated; a place where everyone contributes to each other's growth and healing.

Finding Effective Exercises for Personal Needs

To overcome barriers to somatic healing, it helps to understand your unique patterns and responses. Start by noticing what happens in your body during moments of stress or strong emotion: tightness in your shoulders, a racing heart, or shallow breath. Keeping a short journal of these experiences can help you identify what your body needs most from your healing practice.

Healing is an experiment in listening. Try different somatic exercises, like grounding, gentle stretching, mindful breathing, or emotional flow, and note how your body responds. If a practice leaves you feeling calmer or more present, it's worth returning to. If something feels uncomfortable or draining, that's valuable information, too.

To make exploration more engaging, try an activity I call Somatic Roulette. It's a playful way to reconnect with the practices you've already learned in this book while staying open to new discoveries.

Structure of the Game

1. Think about several somatic exercises you've enjoyed or are curious to revisit (for example, grounding breath, mirroring, movement journaling, or mindful walking) and assign each exercise a number.
2. Pick a number, and practice the chosen exercise for 5–15 minutes, giving it your full attention.
3. Afterward, take a moment to reflect: *How do you feel? What sensations did you notice? What surprised you?*

Optional Variations

- Invite a friend to join you and share reflections afterward.
- Choose a theme for the day, like "calm," "energy," or "release," and select exercises that match that focus.

Each time you play, you'll deepen your awareness of which practices best support your needs. Over time, this becomes less about experimenting and more about building a personal toolkit for balance and emotional regulation.

Adapting Somatic Practices to Suit Your Needs and Lifestyle

Not every somatic practice will feel like the perfect fit, and that's completely normal. The key isn't to give up on the ones that don't immediately click, but to find ways to make them work for you. Adapt the pace, setting, or intensity so the practice aligns with your personality, comfort level, and daily rhythm. When you tailor somatic exercises to your lifestyle, they become more sustainable and enjoyable, allowing you to experience their full benefit over time.

Checking In With Yourself

One of the first steps in adapting somatic practices is learning to check in with yourself before you begin. Each day brings its own energy, emotions, and needs, and honoring that variability helps you choose what feels most supportive in the moment. On days when you feel energized, you might be drawn to movement that feels dynamic, like brisk walking, dancing, or light strength training.

When your energy is lower or your emotions feel tender, gentler practices such as stretching, restorative yoga, or slow breathing can offer comfort and balance. By tuning into your body's signals instead of pushing past them, you begin to build a deeper, more compassionate relationship with your own well-being.

By regularly checking in with your body, you begin to notice not just *what* it needs but also *how much* it needs. Some days call for deeper, longer practices, while others simply need a few mindful minutes of movement to reset your energy and focus.

Opting for Short Sessions

A practical way to integrate movement into daily life is through short bursts of activity. These brief sessions do not require a significant time commitment but can still be highly effective. For instance, setting a timer for 5 minutes and doing a quick meditative exercise or grounding practice can invigorate both body and mind. This approach allows for flexibility, meaning that even on busy days, there is room for somatic activity.

Additionally, engaging in these short breaks throughout the day can help maintain energy levels and improve your overall mood. It's about finding little pockets of time to move, which can be infused into daily tasks like taking the stairs instead of the elevator or doing a few stretches during work breaks.

Changing Times and Locations

Additionally, you can experiment with the timing and setting of your exercises. You may prefer morning workouts to start the day with energy, or you might find evening sessions help you unwind. Finding the right environment enhances the somatic experience. A peaceful park, a cozy room, or even an open space at home can make a significant difference. Each setting can impact how you feel while performing the exercises, influencing your motivation and enjoyment.

By embracing a mindset of adaptability, you can make somatic therapy a sustainable part of life. It's vital to remember that the key is not perfection, but rather, progress. Each adaptation is a step toward creating a more personalized routine that enhances your well-being. There is freedom in exploring what feels right in the moment, whether that means trying a new movement, adjusting the intensity, or simply changing the location of your practices.

Furthermore, embracing change in somatic practices as a natural progression builds resilience. As your body ages or circumstances change, the ability to shift your practices accordingly can preserve the joy of movement. Instead of viewing limitations as obstacles, you can see them as opportunities to explore new forms of exercise.

Key Takeaways

- It is common to encounter challenges surrounding somatic therapy, such as the societal stigmas and misunderstandings linked to these practices or not finding techniques that meet your preferences.
- A big part of overcoming these challenges is educating yourself about somatic therapy so you can understand the value of the practices and ways to modify them to suit your lifestyle needs.
- Historically, the medical community has favored methods such as traditional psychotherapy to respond to various physical and mental conditions. However, we're seeing more interest in learning about alternative methods like body-centered therapies.
- By sharing your experiences integrating somatic practices in your life, you can help demystify this healing approach and encourage others to explore somatic practices. These efforts promote broader acceptance of somatic therapy in wellness discussions.

By continuing to share knowledge, stories, and experiences through social media and community networks, we help create a more inclusive space where mind–body healing is seen, respected, and understood. This collective conversation deepens awareness and supports not just individual growth, but a shared evolution toward holistic well-being.

In the next and final chapter, we'll bring everything together with a practical 28-day plan designed to help you combine your favorite somatic exercises into a consistent, enjoyable routine, one that supports lasting balance, connection, and renewal.

11.

Bonus Chapter: The 28-Day Somatic Challenge

What drains your spirit drains your body. What fuels your spirit fuels your body. –Caroline Myss

"

When I began incorporating somatic practices into my own life, I didn't have a plan or structure. I simply started listening, really listening, to what my body was trying to tell me. Some days it asked for stillness, other days for movement. Over time, those small moments of awareness began to change everything.

This 28-day somatic challenge is an invitation for you to experience this same shift. It's a way to bring gentle, intentional practices into your daily routine and notice how they shape your energy, mood, and overall sense of balance. Each day offers a simple prompt or exercise designed to help you reconnect with your body, your emotions, and your inner rhythm.

There's no pressure to get it right. The goal is simply to show up with curiosity, giving yourself the gift of presence. By the end of these four weeks, you'll not only feel more attuned to your body but also more connected to the calm and vitality that come from truly inhabiting yourself.

Creating a Daily Practice Schedule

Starting the 28-day somatic challenge needs more than just enthusiasm; you need a clear plan to stay consistent and make progress. One effective way to do this is to create a visual schedule: a 28-day calendar just for your somatic exercises. This visual guide maps out your journey and helps you build a daily habit that boosts motivation and accountability.

You can check your calendar at the start of each day so you know what you'll do in your somatic practice. It might seem like a small act, but it can motivate you by reminding you of your commitment and showing your progress. Seeing your journey laid out helps you feel more responsible, making it less likely that you'll skip days.

It's also important to set specific times for your practice. In our busy lives, time can slip away if we don't make an effort to plan. Setting aside certain times each day for your somatic exercises can ease feelings of being overwhelmed and help you stick to your commitment. Many find success by fitting these practices into their existing routines—maybe first thing in the morning or as a way to wind down before bed. Whatever time you pick, consistency is key. Your body likes routine, and honoring that can help make the challenge feel like a normal part of your life.

While it might seem strict to plan everything, it's essential to include weekly themes in your focus. These themes keep your practice interesting throughout the 28 days. Each week, focus on a different part of somatic practice. For example, maybe the first week is about breathwork and how breathing affects your body awareness. In the second week, you could explore movement and how it relates to your emotions. Changing your focus regularly keeps your mind curious, which is essential for staying committed long-term.

Be Flexible With Your Practice

Even with a structured plan, being flexible is important for maintaining your practice. Life can be unpredictable, and unexpected things can throw off the best plans. Being flexible lets you adjust instead of seeing changes as failures. If one day doesn't go as planned because of work or family, don't ditch your practice. Move your exercise to a different time or change its intensity to fit your situation. Being adaptable in this way makes the whole experience more in tune with your life.

For example, if you work full-time and feel anxious, a strict schedule might add stress. You might find it helpful to know you can practice during lunch instead of sticking only to evenings. Personalizing your approach supports long-term commitment because it acknowledges that some days will naturally be tougher than others.

Keep in mind, the goal is to integrate somatic exercises into your life easily—creating a routine that feels comfortable and familiar. Establishing a lasting practice means balancing structure with the ability to adjust as needed. Your calendar gives you clarity, setting specific times provides stability, themes keep things engaging, and flexibility ensures you can stick with it over time.

Tips for Staying Motivated

Taking on a 28-day somatic challenge is a big commitment, and staying motivated allows you to see meaningful results. One useful strategy is to create a reward system. When you connect your achievements with things that motivate you, it strengthens your commitment. Rewards don't have to be big; they can be simple things that make you happy. Maybe it's spending time on a favorite hobby or taking a nice walk outside. These rewards can boost your spirits and make it exciting to achieve your future goals.

After completing two weeks of the somatic challenge, treat yourself to something enjoyable—like a special dinner or a relaxing evening with friends. Recognizing and rewarding your progress keeps your enthusiasm alive. Just remember, the rewards should add to your experience instead of becoming distractions; they should enhance the well-being and satisfaction you gain from your progress.

Affirm Yourself Regularly

While external rewards are helpful, internal affirmations are just as important for staying motivated. Positive affirmations can strengthen your belief in yourself and help build resilience over time. By reminding yourself of your abilities and strengths each day, you create a protective mental environment against self-doubt. Consider starting each day with affirmations like, "I can achieve what I set my mind to accomplish" or "Every mindful moment moves me closer to my best self."

These affirmations work best when you repeat them regularly and make them part of your daily routine. You might say them out loud in the morning or write them in a journal. Gradually, they can transform your inner dialogue, which can lead to a growth mindset that prepares you for any challenge.

Linking your reward system to your well-being can also help keep you engaged. This creates a positive cycle where rewards help with your overall growth. For instance, if yoga or meditation lifts your mood, use these as rewards for reaching goals. When you tie physical rewards to emotional well-being, it reinforces the connection between your progress and positive results.

Tracking Your Experiences and Outcomes

Checking your progress is an important tool for growing self-awareness throughout this challenge. A simple way to do this is through daily journaling prompts. Writing in a journal encourages you to explore your thoughts more deeply, giving you better insight into your emotions. Journaling isn't just a way to keep records; it's a reflective practice that helps you process emotions and gain insights.

To support this reflective journey, using progress tracking tools gives you a visual way to see your development. Whether simple charts or more advanced apps, these tools give you real proof of your transformation. Seeing your progress visually can be very motivating. It turns your personal development into something solid, enhancing your sense of achievement and encouraging you to keep going. Regularly updating these tools allows you to follow your growth path, boosting your motivation and helping you notice subtle changes that might go unseen.

Noticing patterns in your emotions or physical feelings is important in becoming more mindful of your body. As you document your experiences daily, you may see recurring themes. For example, you might notice tension often builds in your shoulders when you're stressed or that certain thoughts trigger specific physical reactions.

Recognizing these patterns strengthens your connection with your body, helping you to pay attention to how your feelings show up physically. Essentially, you'll notice that with greater mental and physical awareness, you can handle stress better and build a healthier relationship with your mind and body.

Collecting data during this process gives you valuable information for adjusting your practice to meet your personal needs. This data also serves as a foundation for tailoring your somatic practices. For example, if you find yourself anxious before a certain activity, you can change your routine to include calming exercises beforehand. Adjusting your practices according to what you learn about yourself ensures they stay relevant and effective.

As you move forward, you'll likely find recurring emotional or physical patterns. These can be valuable learning experiences and signs of progress. Recognizing that an energy boost can follow vulnerability or that deep breathing eases anxiety can help you respond more effectively to similar situations later.

By acknowledging these patterns, through meditation, breathing exercises, or other somatic techniques, you learn to respond thoughtfully rather than react impulsively, building proactive coping skills that enhance emotional resilience.

Collecting information about your somatic journey goes beyond tracking numbers or routines, it's about noticing the patterns, lessons, and wisdom your body reveals over time. Think of it as creating your own library of self-knowledge. Each note or reflection becomes a clue about what supports your well-being and what might need adjusting.

As you learn more about yourself, let this awareness guide how you refine your somatic practices. When your routines evolve in response to lived experience, they become more meaningful and aligned with your natural rhythm, leading to steady and lasting shifts in both mental and physical health.

As your awareness deepens, having a simple way to track your experiences can help you stay consistent and notice patterns. Recording your reflections not only keeps you accountable but also reveals how small, steady efforts create meaningful change.

28-Day Somatic Challenge Tracker Example

How to use this tracker:

✓ Check off each day's practice to build consistency.
✓ Take a moment to reflect and notice your experiences.
✓ Adjust as needed—flexibility is key!

Week 1: Breath Awareness & Grounding

This first week centers on slowing down, reconnecting with your breath, and cultivating awareness of how your body feels in the present moment. Think of it as setting a foundation, before movement and emotion can flow freely, the body needs to feel safe and supported.

Focus: Deep breathing, grounding exercises, and body awareness.

Day	Activity Completed? (✓)	Notes (How did you feel today?)
1		
2		
3		
4		
5		
6		
7		

End-of-week reflection: Take a moment to look back on the week as a whole. *What changes did you notice in your breath and body awareness? Were there particular moments that felt grounding or restorative?*

Week 2: Movement & Emotional Connection

In the second week, you'll begin to deepen the mind–body relationship by introducing more movement into your daily practice. This is where the awareness you built through grounding and breath in Week 1 starts to take shape. Movement allows emotions that have been stored or suppressed to surface safely and flow through you, rather than staying trapped in the body.

Focus: Explore movement-based exercises like stretching, intuitive dancing, or walking meditation.

Day	Activity Completed? (✓)	Notes (How did you feel today?)
8		
9		
10		
11		
12		
13		
14		

End-of-week reflection: Consider what your body taught you through movement this week. *What insights or changes stood out as you stayed consistent with your practice?*

____

____

____

____

Week 3: Sensory Awareness & Self-Compassion

This week invites you to slow down and connect more deeply with your senses. By bringing awareness to touch, taste, sound, and sight, you begin to reawaken the body's natural intelligence and its capacity for calm. Sensory practices ground you in the present moment while cultivating gentleness toward yourself, an essential part of healing and integration.

Focus: Engage your senses, try mindful touch, eating, or listening exercises.

Day	Activity Completed? (✓)	Notes (How did you feel today?)
15		
16		
17		
18		
19		
20		
21		

End-of-week reflection: Consider which of your senses felt most alive and what that experience revealed to you about presence and embodiment.

____

____

____

Week 4: Integration & Flexibility

This final week brings together everything you've practiced so far: breath, movement, sensory awareness, and compassion. Integration means weaving these insights into your everyday life, allowing somatic awareness to become a natural part of who you are. Flexibility is equally important; your body and emotions will continue to change, and your practices can evolve right alongside them.

Focus: Incorporate what you've learned into daily routines and adapt practices as needed.

Day	Activity Completed? (✓)	Notes (How did you feel today?)
22		
23		
24		
25		
26		
27		
28		

End-of-week reflection: Consider what inner or outer shift supported you most this week. *How did this change influence your overall sense of grounding and well-being?*

____

____

____

As you complete this 28-day journey, take a moment to honor your commitment to self-awareness and healing. Every checkmark, reflection, and moment of presence has helped strengthen the connection between your body, mind, and spirit. Remember that this challenge isn't an ending, it's a beginning. Let the insights you've gained continue to guide your days, reminding you that your body is a wise and trusted ally on your path to balance, resilience, and renewal.

Key Takeaways

- This chapter has explored how to create a practical schedule that balances accountability and flexibility. By making a visual calendar and setting specific times, we've built a foundation that supports consistency without being overly strict.
- Weekly themes keep your practices engaging and help you integrate them into the flow of life. Being able to adjust your plans when needed allows you to stick with your commitment even when challenges arise.
- By thoughtfully organizing your 28-day journey, you tap into the connection between discipline and flexibility, allowing for personal transformation. The combination of structure, curiosity, and self-kindness promotes growth throughout the challenge, making it an enjoyable part of your daily routine.

Remember, flexibility isn't a barrier to progress; it strengthens it by recognizing life's unpredictability. Each step you take in this journey is evidence of your growth and the positive relationship you're building with yourself.

Conclusion

Our body and mind have the capacity to heal themselves if we allow them to rest. Stopping, calming, and resting are preconditions for healing. –Thich Nhat Hanh

“

When I began my own healing journey, I didn’t fully understand how much my body was trying to speak to me. Like many, I carried years of emotion: grief, exhaustion, and unspoken fears, without realizing how they were shaping my health and happiness. What I’ve come to learn is that our bodies remember everything, but they also hold an extraordinary capacity to heal when given care and attention. This book was written to share what I’ve learned along the way, to offer you a path toward listening inward, reconnecting with yourself, and trusting the wisdom already within you.

You’ve probably noticed how stress shows up physically: tight shoulders, fatigue, or lingering aches that seem to have no cause. These sensations are the body’s way of speaking the language of emotion. When you start noticing these signs and respond with curiosity instead of frustration, you begin to bridge the gap between how you feel and how you function. This awareness becomes the first step toward aligning your emotional and physical well-being.

Awareness, though, is only the beginning. Healing deepens through small, consistent acts of care; moments when you choose to breathe, stretch, or slow down instead of pushing through. Much like tending a garden, it’s the steady attention that allows growth to take root.

Even a few minutes of somatic practice each day can shift how you relate to yourself, bringing calm where there was tension and steadiness where there was strain. These moments build upon each other, creating a foundation of strength that supports you long after the practice itself ends.

Throughout these chapters, you've explored many ways to reconnect with your body and emotions. Yet the most important truth is that your healing will never look exactly like anyone else's. What works for one person may not fit for another, and that's okay. Your body knows what it needs. The more you listen and adapt, the more personal and powerful your journey becomes. Each practice you choose is an act of agency; a way of saying, *"I trust myself enough to take part in my own healing."*

Healing also thrives in connection. Having others who understand what you're experiencing can make all the difference. Community reminds us that we don't have to carry everything alone. Whether you join a somatic support group, work with a therapist, or simply share your reflections with a trusted friend, these connections offer strength, understanding, and encouragement. In community, you'll find people who will witness your story with compassion and celebrate your progress alongside you.

As you reach the end of this book, remember that healing isn't a finish line; it's a lifelong relationship with yourself. The mind-body connection offers a way to navigate life with more clarity and kindness. It teaches you to recognize your body's signals and respond with care, to rest when needed, and to move when your energy calls for release. Within you is the capacity to transform pain into understanding and to meet your experiences with renewed strength.

There will still be days that feel heavy or uncertain, but those moments no longer have to define you. The more you return to your body's wisdom, the more you'll realize that resilience lives inside you. Healing is a process of remembering who you are beneath the layers of survival: steady, capable, and whole.

As you move forward, let these practices weave naturally into your daily rhythm. Use them as touchstones in times of stress and as rituals of connection in moments of stillness. The consistency you build will nurture peace in both mind and body, helping you meet life's challenges from a place of calm awareness. You are no longer defined by what you've endured, but by how deeply you choose to care for yourself now.

Somatic work taught me how to listen: to my breath, my heartbeat, my fatigue, my tears. It showed me that the body speaks long before the mind catches up, and that safety, softness, and strength all begin there. Writing this book was not only a way to share what I've learned, but also a continuation of my own healing. Each chapter was written with the hope that it might serve as a lantern for someone else walking through their own darkness.

If these pages have helped you pause, breathe, or reconnect with yourself in even the smallest way, then the intention behind this work has been fulfilled. Healing is deeply personal, but it is also something we can witness and nurture in one another. My wish is that you continue to honor your body's wisdom and treat it as both sacred and trustworthy; a guide that knows how to lead you home.

References

Amos, T. (n.d.). *Tori Amos quotes*. BrainyQuote. https://www.brainyquote.com/quotes/tori_amos_183441

Bishop, D. (2021, November 24). *Somatic awareness: 5 activities to increase somatic awareness - oasis recovery center*. Oasis Recovery Center. https://www.or-nc.com/somatic-awareness-5-activities-to-increase-somatic-awareness/

Brom, D., Stokar, Y., Lawi, C., Nuriel-Porat, V., Ziv, Y., Lerner, K., & Ross, G. (2017). Somatic experiencing for posttraumatic stress disorder: A randomized controlled outcome study. *Journal of Traumatic Stress, 30*(3), 304–312. https://doi.org/10.1002/jts.22189

Buddha. (n.d.). *Buddha quotes*. QuoteFancy. https://quotefancy.com/quote/1705485/Buddha-Our-sorrows-and-wounds-are-healed-only-when-we-touch-them-with-compassion

Caporuscio, J. (2024, September 9). Grounding techniques for anxiety, PTSD, and trauma. *Medical News Today*. https://www.medicalnewstoday.com/articles/grounding-techniques

Chödrön, P. (n.d.). *Pema Chödrön quotes*. Goodreads. https://www.goodreads.com/quotes/506874-you-are-the-sky-everything-else-it-s-just-the

Cohen, I. S. (2023, November 13). Understanding Bowen family systems theory. *Psychology Today*. https://www.psychologytoday.com/za/blog/your-emotional-meter/202311/understanding-bowen-family-systems-theory

Cronkleton, E. (2024, May 17). *10 breathing exercises to try when you're feeling stressed*. Healthline. https://www.healthline.com/health/breathing-exercise

Faust, P. (2020, December 11). *Laughter yoga - huh?* LinkedIn. https://www.linkedin.com/pulse/laughter-yoga-huh-patricia-faust/

Gibran, K. (n.d.). *Khalil Gibran quotes*. BrainyQuote. https://www.brainyquote.com/quotes/khalil_gibran_386848

Giraud, M., Javadi, A.-H., Lenatti, C., Allen, J., Tamè, L., & Nava, E. (2024). The role of the somatosensory system in the feeling of emotions: a neurostimulation study. *Social Cognitive and Affective Neuroscience, 19*(1). https://doi.org/10.1093/scan/nsae062

Gould, W. R. (2024, March 21). *What is a sound bath?* Verywell Mind. https://www.verywellmind.com/what-are-sound-baths-4783501

Hanh, T. N. (1998, May 1). *Thich Nhat Hanh quotes.* Goodreads. https://www.goodreads.com/quotes/10702524-calming-allows-us-to-rest-and-resting-is-a-precondition

Hesse, H. (n.d.). *Hermann Hesse quotes.* Goodreads. https://www.goodreads.com/quotes/7540208-within-you-there-is-a-stillness-and-a-sanctuary-to

Holzer, P. (2022). Gut signals and gut feelings: Science at the interface of data and beliefs. *Frontiers in Behavioral Neuroscience, 16.* https://doi.org/10.3389/fnbeh.2022.929332

How does trauma affect the parasympathetic nervous system? (2020, March 2). Mental Health Services. https://www.mhs-dbt.com/blog/parasympathetic-nervous-system-and-trauma/

Kabat-Zinn, J. (n.d.). *Jon Kabat-Zinn quotes.* Goodreads. https://www.goodreads.com/quotes/331826-you-can-t-stop-the-waves-but-you-can-learn-to

Lindberg, S. (2023, November 22). *What is dance therapy?* Verywell Mind. https://www.verywellmind.com/dance-therapy-and-eating-disorder-treatment-5094952

Mahamenan, A. (2024, May 30). *Bharatanatyam: Does this expressive form of Indian classical dancing put the mind to ease?* St. George's University of London. https://www.sgul.ac.uk/about/our-education-centres/centre-for-innovation-and-development-in-education/inclusive-education/inclusive-education-blog/Bharatanatyam-Does-this-expressive-form-of-Indian-classical-dancing-put-the-mind-to-ease

Murakami, H. (1987, September 4). *Haruki Murakami quotes.* Goodreads. https://www.goodreads.com/quotes/338350-what-happens-when-people-open-their-hearts-they-get-better

Myss, C. (2011, December 1). *Carolyn Myss quotes.* Goodreads. https://www.goodreads.com/quotes/833002-what-drains-your-spirit-drains-your-body-what-fuels-your

Newton, C. (2011, July). *The five communication styles.* Claire Newton. https://www.clairenewton.co.za/my-articles/the-five-communication-styles.html

Orzechowska, A., Maruszewska, P., & Gałecki, P. (2021). Cognitive behavioral therapy of patients with somatic symptoms—diagnostic and therapeutic difficulties. *Journal of Clinical Medicine, 10*(14), 3159. https://doi.org/10.3390/jcm10143159

Ott, S. L. (2023, March 9). *Mind-body connection: Somatic therapy and mindfulness.* Dr. Sophia Lin Ott. https://www.drsophialinott.com/blog/2023/3/9/mind-body-connection-somatic-therapy-and-mindfulness

Rapkoch, K. (2024, December 9). *Somatic breathwork: A guide to nervous system reset.* Re-Origin. https://www.re-origin.com/articles/somatic-breathwork

Remen, R. N. (n.d.). *Rachel Naomi Remen quotes.* Goodreads. https://www.goodreads.com/quotes/491458-healing-may-not-be-so-much-about-getting-better-as

Rousseau, D. (2023, December 13). *The effect of trauma on the brain.* Boston University. https://sites.bu.edu/daniellerousseau/2023/12/13/the-effect-of-trauma-on-the-brain/

Rumi. (n.d.). *Rumi quotes.* Goodreads. https://www.goodreads.com/quotes/9726-your-task-is-not-to-seek-for-love-but-merely

Salamon, M. (2023, July 7). *What is somatic therapy?* Harvard Health. https://www.health.harvard.edu/blog/what-is-somatic-therapy-202307072951

Schmitt, C. M., & Schoen, S. (2022). Interoception: A multi-sensory foundation of participation in daily life. *Frontiers in Neuroscience, 16*. https://doi.org/10.3389/fnins.2022.875200

Scott, E. (2024, February 12). *What is body scan meditation?* Verywell Mind. https://www.verywellmind.com/body-scan-meditation-why-and-how-3144782

Singh, K., Saran, S., & Jerard, P. (n.d.). *Balancing your brain in yoga class*. Aura Wellness Center. https://aurawellnesscenter.com/2023/04/19/balancing-your-brain-in-yoga-class/

Stoyanova, D. (n.d.). *Darina Stoyanova quotes.* Pinterest. https://mx.pinterest.com/pin/762304674436869673/

Stubbe, D. E. (2018). Complementary and alternative medicine: If you don't ask, they won't tell. *Focus: Journal of Life Long Learning in Psychiatry, 16*(1), 60–62. https://doi.org/10.1176/appi.focus.20170052

Tank, A. (2024, November 5). *How I use habit stacking to build better habits into my workday*. Medium. https://medium.com/swlh/how-i-use-habit-stacking-to-build-better-habits-into-my-workday-d550fb66deed

Yang, I. (2024, May 2). *You deserve a moment of relaxation. these 7 yoga poses can help give you that.* Peloton. https://www.onepeloton.com/blog/yoga-for-relaxation

Made in the USA
Monee, IL
04 November 2026

67384750R00105